PUSH BACK

PUSH
BACK

Guilt in the Age of Natural Parenting

Amy B. Tuteur, MD

DEY ST.
AN IMPRINT OF WILLIAM MORROW PUBLISHERS

HarperCollins books may be purchased for educational, business, or sales promotional use. For information please e-mail the Special Markets Department at SPsales @harpercollins.com.

FIRST EDITION

Library of Congress Cataloging-in-Publication Data has been applied for.

ISBN 978-0-06-240734-4

16 17 18 19 20   DIX/RRD   10 9 8 7 6 5 4 3 2 1

For my husband, Michael.
Thirty-five years after our wedding,
I still do!

Contents

Introduction

Several hundred years ago, a famous philosopher said, *"Cogito, ergo sum"* (I think, therefore I am).

My motto is a bit different: *I mother, therefore I am guilty.*

If you are a mother, and chances are that if you are reading this book you are, then this may be your motto too.

My children are grown now, but I have not forgotten the pervasive feeling of guilt that parenting can engender. It has ever been thus. I can't help you with most of the guilt that comes naturally with mothering—the guilt over school choice, screen time, sibling rivalry, or discipline styles—but there is one area in which I can offer comfort. There is *no reason* to feel guilty about any childbirth choices or choices of early infancy.

No woman should ever feel guilty about the choices she makes regarding childbirth, breastfeeding, or the manner in which she cares for her baby. Surprised? Unfortunately we live in a society where these fundamental aspects of a woman's life are now an arena where judgment, second-guessing, and guilt reign supreme. It is no longer enough to give birth to a healthy baby and to care for that baby, providing food, warmth, and tenderness. Now all of these acts must be done, in many circles, in ways decreed "correct" by the natural parenting industry.

Where did this industry that dictates the behaviors of millions of women come from?

Surprisingly, the currently popular philosophies of natural childbirth, lactivism, and attachment parenting are based on nothing more than the personal beliefs of a few individuals, most of them men. To my mind, though, the most damaging aspect of this paradigm is that the judgment and guilt surrounding childbirth and child care are heaped upon women most often by other women.

I am an obstetrician and the mother of four children. When I stopped practicing obstetrics, I became a writer, focused of course on women and childbirth. Along the way I saw that there needed to be a voice of reason in the wilds of the Internet focused on mothers and childbirth. So I have spent the last twenty years becoming "She Who Must Not Be Named," Enemy Number One of the Natural Parenting Industry.

Why? Because I have made it my mission to help women escape the feelings of guilt about their birth experience that trap them long after their children are born. I challenge the popular notions out there that are so often rooted in pseudoscience. I offer comfort to expectant and new mothers as they face the difficult task of caring for a newborn while simultaneously listening to a cacophony of voices telling them how to have their babies, how to feed them, how to hold them, and that if they don't follow these edicts, their babies will not thrive and become successful adults. I've used science, common sense, and kindness to dispel what I see as the myths miring women in despair. I've poked holes in the theories of the natural parenting proponents, and in the process I've made some enemies, but I've made a lot more women feel a lot better.

Push Back is my boldest statement yet, and it represents how my own thinking on this topic has evolved over the years. Initially I was simply bewildered by the ways in which my patients tormented themselves. After delivering a beautiful healthy baby to a joyous healthy mother, I would visit her the next day in the hospital and find her tearful over her "failure." Instead of enjoying the miracle of her new child, she would be berating herself that she had "given in" and gotten an epidural for pain relief. Or perhaps she would have concluded that her C-section reflected the fact that her body was "broken." There was a myriad of if-onlys. If only she hadn't agreed to the postterm induction; if only she had trusted birth more. Sometimes I wondered if the process of birth was more important than the baby itself.

When I was a practicing obstetrician, I spent a lot of time correcting the misinformation of natural childbirth advocates and comforting women who'd had healthy babies but still felt guilty for not "achieving" a vaginal birth or a birth without pain relief. Though I was aware of the emotional response from my bedside visits, it took years of blogging about the subject, corresponding with mothers, and arguing with activists to appreciate the true depth, breadth, and prevalence of misinformation coming from the natural parenting movement, and how this has come to blight the experience of mothering infants for so many.

Twenty years ago, when I began writing on the Web, I thought that the problem could be solved with more and better information. Most of what passes for knowledge within the natural childbirth, lactivist, and natural parenting communities is flat out false. Yet simply correcting the plethora of falsehoods seemed to be fruitless. I came to understand that natural childbirth, lactivism, and attachment parenting actually *are* about privileging the process over the outcome.

Natural childbirth, lactivism, and attachment parenting are highly stylized, profoundly idealized representations of parenting. How do we know that they are idealized? Primarily it's because the scientific evidence does not support most of their central tenets. That's not to say that natural parenting advocates don't believe in science; they do and they invoke science a lot. However, a close examination reveals that they often subvert the scientific evidence to arrive at predetermined conclusions.

Why would anyone want to subvert the scientific evidence on childbirth, breastfeeding, and attachment parenting? Because each of these ideas has morphed into businesses, complete with trade unions, lobbying groups, and brilliant marketing. Simply put, misinformation is being promoted by birth and breastfeeding professionals, as well as parenting gurus, as a way to make money. These factions portray doctors as the enemy, and their primary product has become distrust of the medical profession. They created alternate worlds of internal legitimacy in the same way that creationists and anti-vaccine activists have done before them, complete with books, journals, conferences, and certifications to signify "expertise." The Internet has been their greatest enabler, allowing women to "research" parenting decisions without ever leaving a massive echo chamber.

There's far more than money at stake. Beliefs about women and their role in society undergird natural parenting. It seems to me to be more than coincidence that natural childbirth, breastfeeding, and natural parenting share a variety of disturbing characteristics. All impose an inordinate amount of work and pain on women, and all ostensibly exclude fathers and other family members, making women not merely the primary caregivers but the only acceptable caregivers a majority of the time. And by requiring intense around-the-clock effort, they make it nearly impossible for women who want or need something in addition to mothering (a job, a career, free time) to be "good" mothers. It all seems suspiciously like the classic ploy to control and judge women by the performance of their reproductive organs.

When I dove deeper, I was not surprised to find that most of these movements were created or promulgated by elderly white men. Advocates represent natural childbirth, lactivism, and attachment parenting as the ultimate expressions of parental love, combining scientific evidence with maternal devotion, feminism, and respect for maternal choice. The reality is far different. These philosophies that gather under the rubric of natural parenting put forth a pro-woman agenda but in fact are quite the opposite. In this book, I will show the evolution of each of the aspects of natural parenting—natural childbirth, lactivism, and attachment parenting—from their origins to the big businesses they are today, from a search for authentic experiences to a prescribed experience that relegates women back into old-fashioned roles prescribed by gender.

Divided into three sections, *Push Back* tackles the natural parenting industry from all sides, hopefully alleviating the guilt so many women unnecessarily face, revealing it to readers as the damaging, sometimes dangerous construct I think it is.

THE SCIENCE

Why is there such a wide gulf between obstetricians (most of whom these days are women) and the proponents of natural childbirth? It's because natural childbirth is not based on science. From "birth is safe" to "interventions are bad" to "C-sections are almost never necessary," the central tenets of natural childbirth are contradicted by the preponderance of scientific evidence. We will also consider lactivism and attachment parenting. They often go hand in hand with the philosophy of natural childbirth, and women who feel guilty that they "failed" at birth are often determined, if not desperate, to succeed at the other two, at any cost.

THE INDUSTRY

If natural parenting does not comport with the scientific evidence, how has it become embedded in the conventional wisdom of contemporary parenting? The reason is that entire industries profit from it. Midwives and doulas derive a substantial proportion of their income from convincing women that natural childbirth is best. The jobs of lactation consultants depend on convincing women to breastfeed. Innumerable courses, workshops, and websites all derive their income from natural childbirth. "Birth workers" and lactivists have organized themselves into groups that lobby on their behalf, and a variety of nonprofit organizations exist to promote natural childbirth and lobby for it in the halls of state legislatures and Congress. This is a large, politically powerful, and lucrative industry.

THE PHILOSOPHY

For most of human history, women have been reduced to their uteruses, vaginas, and breasts. The natural childbirth theorists, as well as many lactivists and attachment parenting advocates, continue to reduce women to uteruses, vaginas, and breasts, insisting that how they use those body parts determines their worth as human beings.

Ironically, parenting advocates often invoke the language of "choice" to promote natural childbirth, and lactivism, assuming that if a woman has the power of choice, it is automatically a feminist gesture. But natural parenting advocates in fact do not promote choice; they promote their *specific* choices and try to shame those women who choose differently.

In other words, these movements are judgmental and anti-woman.

My goal with this book is to release women from the guilt trap created by the natural parenting industry and to begin a dialogue based in reclaiming safety, common sense, and joy, so that women can mother in whatever way best meets their personal needs and the needs of their families.

I've learned over the years that claims like mine require a presentation of my bona fides. No, not my college and medical school training, nor my years of internship, residency, and private practice. I'm talking about my bona fides as a mother, since opponents try to dismiss my presentation of the scientific evidence as sour grapes from someone who couldn't muster the requisite "achievements." I have four children (all adult or college age now). All were born vaginally after easy labors, two with epidurals and two without. I breastfed all four children until they weaned themselves. I carried them around all the time and my husband and I had an "open bed" policy that resulted in many nights of a small child splayed in the middle of our bed and the two of us trying to sleep while clinging to the edge, hoping not to fall out.

In contemporary parlance, I would be described as an attachment parent, though that terminology did not exist when my children were small. But if I've learned anything from practicing medicine and from more than twenty-five years as a mother, it is this: What works for me and my family is not necessarily what is best for anyone else. The experience of practicing medicine allowed me to meet people from every walk of life, every ethnic group, and every culture. I learned that there are lots of ways to successfully raise children. That conviction has only been strengthened by watching the children of my friends and the friends of my children grow up. Many were raised very differently, and they turned out to be happy, confident, accomplished young adults.

A NOTE ABOUT MIDWIVES

I have always worked with certified nurse-midwives (CNMs), the most highly educated, best-trained midwives in the world. The CNMs I worked with were extremely competent and deeply compassionate. Although they may have held strong views on what a "good birth" meant for them personally, I never saw them substitute their beliefs for a laboring woman's own experience.

Unfortunately, in the last twenty years, midwifery has been progressively radicalized, particularly in the UK and Australia and among the midwifery leaders and theorists in the United States. They have promoted themselves as the "guardians" of normal birth, instead of the guardians of the health and well-being of mothers and babies. Many believe they know better than women themselves whether those women need pain relief, should have interventions, or want a vaginal birth. In short, they have replaced the medical patriarchy with the matriarchy.

It is this radicalized view of the midwives and their role that I take to task in this book.

*

As I noted above, to hear natural childbirth advocates and lactivists tell it, the entire story of mothering can be reduced to three body parts: the uterus, the vagina, and breasts. I've been thinking about how I have mothered my four children over the past twenty-eight years, and it seems as if I have used just about every part of my body.

Arms: I used my arms a lot, not just to carry my children, although I carried them quite a bit when they were small. I used my arms primarily to embrace them. Hugs are the appropriate response in times of both happiness and sadness, or for no better reason than to be close. I cannot count the times I hugged my children, and even now, when they are adults, I still do.

Hands: I think I spent ten solid years holding hands. Holding toddlers' hands when they learned to walk. Holding hands crossing the street and in the parking lot. Holding hands just because it is fun to hold hands.

I also used my hands to sew clothes for my children, to fill out a million permission sheets for field trips, to feel foreheads for temperatures, and to help with a billion school projects. (If anyone needs pipe cleaners, I still have hundreds!)

Lips: I kissed my children over and over and over again. I kissed boo-boos. I kissed to check for fevers. I kissed for no better reason than I loved to kiss them. Of course there were years I had to lay off the kissing because public kissing was just too embarrassing for teenagers, but those years are over now, and I can kiss them again, at least when I'm greeting them.

Legs: I walked miles holding fretful infants in the middle of the night; shopping for clothes and shoes and toys; tramping out to baseball fields, football fields, soccer fields, and basketball courts to cheer my children on.

Mouth: I used it to tell my children that I loved them, but I also used it to advocate for them, to seek out appropriate evaluation and therapy for learning disabilities, to explain them to teachers, to explain life's lessons to them, and to praise them when they did something amazing, which was often.

My entire body: Is there anything that gives comfort like a mother's body? It provides comfort when you are awake sitting near your children, and even when you are asleep lying next to them in bed after a nightmare.

Brain: I thought about my children constantly, when I was with them and when I was not. I taught them facts and I taught them morals. I worried when they were little; I worried when they were teenagers; and I still worry now. I shared my views on how they should treat others and how they should be proud of themselves (or not, as the case warranted). I conveyed my religious beliefs and my political views. I planned for them, I brainstormed with them, and I hoped desperately that I could give them what they needed to be happy and healthy and to reach their full potential.

Last, but not least, I used **my heart**. Of course I don't mean my physical heart, although it sometimes felt like it when they were hurt or disappointed. I am referring to my metaphorical heart. I loved and I still love my children more than life itself and I have tried to convey that to them. They and their father are the most important people in the universe as far as I am concerned, and it is my deepest wish that they know it and feel it.

Yes, my children grew in my uterus. Yes, they transited my vagina when they were born. Yes, I nourished them with my breasts, but I don't think that made much difference to who they are and to how I love them. I would gladly have had C-sections if there had been even the slightest chance that they were at risk during birth. I would have happily supplemented with formula if I hadn't been lucky to produce enough milk. My children don't remember those days, and frankly, they couldn't care less.

That's fine with me. Those body parts are not the ones that I want my children to think of when they think of me. I want them to remember holding hands when they were little, countless hugs and endless kisses. I hope they remember my physical presence beside them when they were sick, next to them in bed when they had bad dreams and in the bleachers or the audience for sports and plays and graduations.

I, like most women, mother with my entire body. Isn't that what good mothers do?

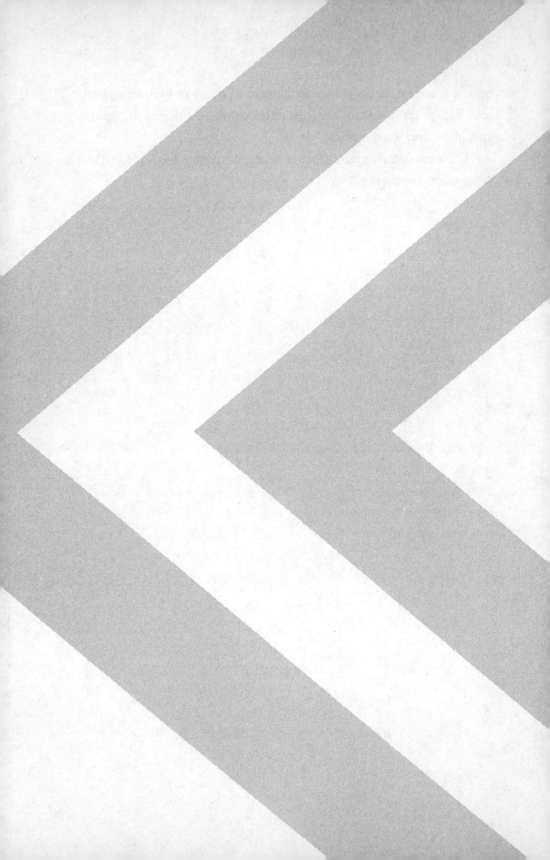

PART 1

SUBVERTING THE SCIENCE

< 1 >

Natural Childbirth Is Nothing Like Childbirth in Nature

I t's a privilege to be an obstetrician and to be invited to witness one of the most important events in the life of a family.

I've been present at some spectacular grand entrances: babies born in the emergency room, quadruplets, and a woman who gave birth without knowing she was pregnant (twice!). Most end happily no matter how dramatic they are. I can vividly recall a woman who came in near her due date bleeding very heavily. At the time, I thought I had never seen so much blood. We rushed to the operating room and delivered a rather stunned newborn by C-section. With a little help from the neonatologist, he was fine. I felt traumatized and I imagined the mother did too. When I visited her on rounds the next morning, I asked if she had any concerns. Indeed she did! She had ordered toast for breakfast and got an English muffin instead. She was incensed.

Although obstetrics is generally a happy profession, there are moments of profound sadness. I remember the identical twins whose umbilical cords became tangled in their mother's uterus and the tragic result. I will never forget the baby who was transverse for most of the pregnancy; he finally turned before his mother arrived in labor, but he did not survive the process. And I'm still profoundly saddened when I think about the young couple who came in in labor with their first child on Christmas Day. They were giddy about having a Christmas baby. Then the nurse couldn't find the baby's heartbeat, and after checking an ultrasound, I had to tell them the devastating news that the baby had died.

Obstetrics can be filled with pure adrenaline-driven moments: the baby who is born not breathing but soon gasps for those first breaths; the baby whose shoulders get stuck and requires extra help coming through the birth canal; the baby whose heart rate drops during labor and stays down for many minutes as we run to the operating room to rescue her. Forget race car driving; obstetrics has more thrills and chills.

I never truly realized how many women believe that childbirth is inherently safe, that a healthy baby is virtually guaranteed, that the worst thing that can happen is getting the wrong breakfast order. It wasn't until I became a blogger that I learned why there is such a gulf between obstetricians' experiences and patients' expectations.

I heard from women like Sarah:

I was raised in the shadow of the story of my mother's successful unmedicated births and how she refused interventions (including ultrasounds) from medical professionals because she wanted to do things naturally and safely. From elementary school on I knew that I wanted to—in fact, needed to—have an unmedicated birth because that was clearly the best and safest way to do it.

Fast-forward to 2010, when I was pregnant with my first (and only) child. I planned to deliver in a hospital with an OB (as had my mother) but was extremely nervous to do so after reading things like Ina May's books and anything from Henci Goer that I could find. I had developed a birth plan asking for nearly no interventions and felt nervous but positive about my upcoming unmedicated hospital birth.

I was devastated when my low-risk pregnancy quickly morphed into high-risk pregnancy in the last trimester.

Why wasn't Sarah prepared for the possibility of developing complications? Had she been led to believe that her birth would and should be simple, easy, and safe? And when things didn't go according to plan, why was that cause for devastation? These are the questions that I wrestle with every day. What is leading women to have unrealistic expectations of what the birth process really is?

Childbirth Without Fear [1] is the book that started it all. Written by Grantly Dick-Read in 1942, this text is widely viewed as the foundational document of the natural childbirth movement. An international bestseller, the book and its message have been embraced by subsequent generations of women. Most of today's proponents of the natural birth ideas set forth in this pre–World War II book aren't aware that its author, while an obstetrician, was also a religious evangelical who believed in the spiritual significance of motherhood. According to Dick-Read, childbirth revealed God's presence. He was also a eugenicist whose philosophies about race and gender had a profound impact on his medical practice and would be viewed today as backward, at best.

Obsessed with the notion that white women of the "better" classes were ignoring their duty to reproduce in favor of pursuing political and economic equality, Grantly Dick-Read feared a decline in the white birthrate. Women must be socialized to return to the home, he insisted, or the white race risked "race suicide." He wrote:

> Woman fails when she ceases to desire the children for
> which she was primarily made. Her true emancipation
> lies in freedom to fulfill her biological purposes.[2]

Part of the problem with the declining birthrate of white babies, Dick-Read felt, was that women curtailed their childbearing due to fear of labor pain. Unlike their "primitive" (read, black) sisters—who were described by other eugenicists as "hypersexual" and had easy, painless labor—"overcivilized" white women had shriveled ovaries, suffered from hysteria (a malady originating in the uterus; *hyster* is Latin for uterus), and had painful labors.

White women, he wrote, had been socialized to give birth in pain, through the fear-tension-pain cycle. Labor, he believed, is not intrinsically painful. Women experienced pain in labor only because they had been taught to anticipate and fear pain; the fear led them to tightening up (tension), and the tension caused the pain. In other words, the pain felt during labor was not real physical pain, but was imagined—and therefore women could also be socialized to give birth without pain. This is the purported "science" that Dick-Read cited for his theories, but his fear-tension-pain cycle was fabricated. As we will see, labor is intrinsically painful for the exact same reasons that passing a kidney stone is intrinsically painful!

In the Dick-Read school of natural childbirth, labor pain served a dual purpose. It was punishment for women who had dared to become "overcivilized" and glaring evidence that women had veered from their "true purpose," that of motherhood. This view reflected the anxieties of social Darwinists and eugenicists as women sought to take their place in the larger society with equal rights such as the right to vote. Victorian and Edwardian physicians and scientists strongly believed that there were fundamental differences between the sexes and the races that led to the ultimate superiority of the white male.

According to Dick-Read, "the mother is the factory, and by education and care she can be made more efficient in the art of motherhood."[3]

A woman's body as a factory? Is this the Old Testament? It is hard to believe that this book launched and remains the bible for the contemporary natural childbirth movement, a movement now comprised largely of educated women who consider themselves both liberated and informed.

Similarly, there were motivations beyond the aid of women involved in the development of Lamaze—the practice of patterned breathing and relaxation popularized in the 1960s in this country to supposedly reduce feelings of pain in labor. Lamaze was born in the postwar Soviet Union, where leaders tried to make a virtue of necessity: they didn't have the painkillers available to ease the pain of birth.[4]

Soviet leaders of the time recognized that it was politically expedient to trumpet new discoveries and methods as products of great Soviet scientists. In the 1940s, few Soviet scientists had a reputation greater than that of Ivan Pavlov, a physiologist known for his development of the concept of the conditioned reflex. Pavlov had observed that when a bell was consistently rung for dogs before they received food, they became conditioned to associate the ringing of the bell with the presentation of food. So closely did they associate the bell with the food, they began to salivate when the bell rang even before the food appeared (behavior now known as the Pavlovian response).

If dogs could be conditioned to associate a bell with food, doctors reasoned that women could be conditioned to associate patterned breathing with pain relief. Then there would be no need for the unaffordable and inaccessible pain medications found in the bourgeois West. This method was promulgated by Immanuel Velikovsky and was far more successful politically than medically. It was promoted in Europe as a Communist success story: Soviet scientists could relieve pain with methods that were nearly free and therefore accessible to poor women as well as to the rich.

Everyone was happy with the method except the Soviet women on whom it was foisted. They found that it didn't relieve their pain. That's not surprising since it is far easier to condition expectations than to condition effective treatment for pain.

The method became known as Lamaze after 1940 when Fernand Lamaze imported the philosophy to French hospitals run by the Communist Party of France, promoting it as an example of the superiority of Soviet science over bourgeois American science.

But common sense, when applied to these ideas, prevails. Of course "primitive women" from tribal cultures don't have painless labors. Childbirth pain is not caused by fear. And women cannot be socialized or conditioned to give birth without pain. A simple description of female anatomy and of how pain works within the body shows that childbirth is simply physically painful—there is no psychological way around this pain. Therefore many women who attempt to adhere to Grantly Dick-Read's prescription of welcoming childbirth as the true purpose of female existence and "trusting" rather than fearing birth inevitably fail, for his mandate is impossible. So for these women, "childbirth without fear" quickly becomes "childbirth with guilt": guilt about feeling pain in labor, guilt about "giving in" to the relief of painkillers, guilt about the "failure" to give birth naturally.

How did a philosophy based on fabricated claims and designed to manipulate women gain so much traction? The answer is timing. Grantly Dick-Read and Lamaze worked at what was the apogee of paternalism in medicine, when doctors were confident that they knew what was good for patients better than the patients did themselves. Not surprisingly, women came to resent the cavalier way they were treated on maternity wards.

Moreover, childbirth anesthesia, which typically involved unconsciousness, was traditionally reserved for the moment of birth itself, the one moment when women preferred to be awake. There were no epidurals then that could have allowed for pain-less labors with women alert and in control throughout labor and delivery. The philosophy of natural childbirth as put forth by Dick-Reid and Lamaze represented the only way for women to be awake and aware for the births of their children.

Natural childbirth became increasingly popular in the 1970s as Americans came to venerate "experiences" of all kinds for their own intrinsic value. Having an unmedicated vaginal birth "like our foremothers" was portrayed as the ultimate experience and therefore very desirable. The popularity of natural childbirth was further enhanced by the fact that it was initially viewed as trans-gressive and antiauthoritarian.

The belief that childbirth pain is a result of socialization is not the only major misrepresentation on which the philosophy of natural childbirth rests. There are two others: the erroneous claim that anything natural must be safe, and the bedrock assertion of midwives, doulas, and other natural childbirth advocates that childbirth itself is an inherently safe process. Unfortunately, both claims conflict with medical and historical reality.

WHAT IS CHILDBIRTH IN NATURE REALLY LIKE?

There once was a time when all childbirth was natural. There were no C-sections, no Pitocin, and no fetal monitors. All babies were breastfed and mothers carried their babies against their bodies constantly. And in that time gone by, when all women gave birth as nature intended, maternal and perinatal mortality rates were . . . astronomical.

Even as late as the early twentieth century, nearly 1 percent of mothers died in childbirth and 7 percent of babies died within the first month. Graveyards were filled with tiny headstones. However, in the past hundred years, since the advent of modern obstetrics (and therefore safe C-sections, safer anesthesia, blood banking, antibiotics, and care for preeclampsia and treatment for gestational diabetes), the neonatal mortality rate has dropped 90 percent and the maternal mortality rate has dropped nearly 99 percent.[5]

The fact is that in every time, place, and culture, childbirth is a leading cause of death of young women and the leading cause of death for the entire eighteen years of childhood. There is no more dangerous day for a child than the day of his or her birth. And yet natural childbirth advocates choose to ignore this altogether. How did they get this so wrong? Ironically, the very success of childbirth interventions has allowed for the idealization of birth and set the stage for contemporary advocates of natural childbirth to bemoan the state of childbirth in America. Their bête noire is the "medicalization" of childbirth: the large numbers of C-sections, the rate of interventions, the use of fetal monitoring—all of the practices now employed to keep women and their babies safe. It is the currently incredibly low rates of neonatal and maternal mortality that have allowed natural childbirth advocates to imagine that childbirth is inherently without danger, and that obstetricians are the one who have complicated it and stripped it of its spiritual meaning by the liberal use of technology. The reality is that childbirth is safe *only* because of the liberal use of technology. Natural childbirth advocates long for an imagined past that literally *never* existed.

Natural childbirth now has an almost cult-like status. Celebrities like Gisele Bündchen, Julianne Moore, and Jennifer Connelly wax poetic about the virtues of natural childbirth. Rarely a week goes by without a movie or TV personality boasting about her planned natural birth. It has been broadcast from the powerful viral pulpit of the TED talk, with the mother of the homebirth movement, Ina May Gaskin, recently delivering a TEDx talk called "Reducing Fear of Birth in U.S. Culture." The wonders of natural childbirth have reached a peak as part of the cultural zeitgeist.

THE PALEOFANTASY OF BIRTH

The idealization of childbirth is a result of the contemporary idealization of nature. In direct opposition to the reality of nature "red in tooth and claw," nature is now viewed as not merely benign but perfect. Professor Marlene Zuk, writing in her book *Paleofantasy: What Evolution Really Tells Us About Sex, Diet, and How We Live,* explains that contemporary Americans[6] are fixated on the imagined behavior of our romanticized hunting-and-foraging ancestors. As Zuk notes, contemporary Americans falsely believe that "our bodies and minds evolved under a particular set of circumstances, and in changing those circumstances without allowing our bodies time to evolve in response, we have wreaked the havoc that is modern life." In this fantasy scenario, we would all be happier and healthier if we just lived like our ancient forebears.

Similarly, natural childbirth advocates claim that birth evolved for a hunter-gatherer lifestyle. They insist that using modern technology in childbirth on women evolved for nontechnological birth has wreaked havoc on women and babies. That's why natural childbirth advocates insist that women should give birth "the way nature intended." The aforementioned Ina May Gaskin, arguably the most outspoken midwife in the natural childbirth movement, refers to becoming attuned to the "ancient wisdom of women's bodies" in order to give birth without medical intervention, as if our ancient selves were innately perfect birthing machines with whom we must reconnect.

According to Gaskin:

> The Creator is not a careless mechanic. Human female bodies have the same potential to give birth well as aardvarks, lions, rhinoceri, elephants, moose, and water buffalo.[7]

Why didn't Gaskin invoke more common, domesticated animals like cows, horses, sheep, dogs, and cats?

Perhaps it is because she realizes that anyone with experience caring for farm animals and pets knows that birth complications, and even death, are quite common (horse intrapartum mortality is 13.7 percent[8]; lamb neonatal mortality is 14.3 percent[9]; among dogs 24.6 percent[10] of litters experience at least one death). In other words, even animals are not "perfectly evolved" to give birth. How clever of Gaskin to invoke animals that are exotic to a majority of people so that she can argue that their births are perfect!

Similarly, hunter-gatherers were never "perfectly evolved"; they represented the best adaptations to conditions as they existed at that time. Conditions have changed dramatically over the past 10,000 years, which means that what was good for them has little relevance for what is good for us. There was never a time that women were "perfectly designed" to give birth, because there has never been a time that any species has been perfectly evolved for anything. Moreover—and this is a critical point that is completely ignored by the paleofantasists—we *have* continued to evolve in keeping with our changing environment.

Human beings have the advantage of technology. We can change our environment and ourselves in ways that evolution would never allow. Ten thousand years ago, if a woman began labor with her baby in a persistent transverse (sideways) position, both she and her baby were guaranteed to die a slow, painful death. Today that mother would have a C-section, and both mother and baby would happily survive. Ten thousand years ago, that mother and baby would have been evolutionary losers. Today they are winners, no thanks to adaptation, but to technology.

The currency of evolution is offspring. If your offspring survive to reproduce, your species wins. If they die, you lose. It's that simple. There are no extra points for vaginal birth or breastfeeding or any other attempts to emulate our foremothers. The woman who has lots of children born safely and healthy, even if they are born via C-section and are bottle-fed, but who themselves go on to reproduce, is the winner. That woman is "perfectly designed" for the environment in which we live.

NO, NATURAL IS NOT BETTER

Natural has become a loaded term, one that means better, often more expensive, and therefore accessible only to the privileged. Natural is now a marketing term and often has nothing to do with nature at all. Advertisers employ it. Organic food purveyors rely on it. One of the more amusing examples of this phenomenon is "Simply Natural Cheetos," as if Cheetos were the preferred snack of prehistoric peoples. And this bizarre idea of "natural" is obviously at the heart of natural childbirth advocacy, lactivism, and attachment parenting.

Yet the belief that natural is better has arisen in a society that proves in every possible way that natural is not better. The average human life expectancy in nature is approximately thirty-five years.[11] The average human life expectancy in first-world countries approaches eighty. What has been responsible for the doubling of life expectancy? It is technology, not nature.

Consider the most fundamental of public health advancements: protecting ourselves from harmful pathogens. To do so, we depend on a variety of strategies that aren't natural. Human waste can cause disease that can be averted with sewer systems. Clean water requires purification plants. Millions around the world live without sewer systems and clean water. This state of things is natural, and it's deadly.

How about our efforts to prevent starvation? Farming is not natural; hunting with weapons is not natural; domesticated animals are not natural. Yet all have profoundly improved the viability of human life.

What about efforts to prevent infections or treat illnesses? Cleaning a wound with antiseptic is not natural. Removing an infected appendix is not natural. Insulin injections for diabetes aren't natural, either. Without them, countless millions who live a full life span would be dead.

Innovations don't have to be lifesaving in order to dramatically enhance our lives. Eyeglasses and hearing aids aren't natural at all, but they improve the quality of life for a large part of our population.

Simply put, just about everything that makes our lives cleaner, safer, more comfortable, and longer is not natural.

So why is contemporary society biased toward the natural?

Marketing has played an enormous but largely unappreciated role in promoting "natural" in order to distinguish products in the marketplace. Marketers have woven a fantasy of benevolent "nature" that invariably costs more. Organic food is a big business, but it provides no nutritional benefits. Homeopathic remedies are just bottled water at a premium price. Herbal supplements are expensive, and many don't even contain the active ingredient listed on the label.

Not surprisingly, Americans with the most disposable income have the means to follow these trends. The fact that rich people choose to spend their money on a product makes it that much more desirable to everyone else. Eating organic food has become a status symbol, having an unmedicated birth is a status symbol, and breastfeeding exclusively is a status symbol.

Many American predilections are grounded in economic status, and childbirth is no different. When poor people were thin because they didn't have enough to eat, being overweight was a sign of status. Similarly, when poor people were tanned because they primarily worked outside, white skin was a sign of status. When poor women couldn't afford anesthesia for childbirth, access to anesthesia was a sign of status.

Natural childbirth costs money. A pregnant woman must buy books and hire childbirth educators and doulas. In the case of homebirth, she must pay a midwife, buy a birth kit, and rent a birthing pool. Breastfeeding is a particularly interesting status symbol. Infant formula became popular in the 1950s, in a milieu where technology itself was a status symbol. The rich could afford the "superior" technological wonder of infant formula while the poor had to make do with breastfeeding. Now that most Americans can afford formula, it has become déclassé. Moreover, breastfeeding is much easier for women who have extended maternity leaves, access to an office to pump, or a breadwinner spouse who allows the mother to stay home with her baby indefinitely. It is much easier to breastfeed if you are a corporate CEO than if you are a hotel chambermaid. "Natural" is now the status symbol, which is why breastfeeding is far more prevalent among well-off white women than among the rest of society.

From an objective point of view, there is no evidence that natural is better. As I have noted, nearly everything that has improved our comfort, health, and life expectancy is not natural. Nonetheless, the bias persists that if it is "natural," it must be good even when there is a massive amount of evidence to the contrary, as in the case of childbirth. And of course there is the supreme irony that natural childbirth advocates and lactivists use every technological method at their disposal (the Internet, advertising, and lobbying) in an effort to argue that technology is bad and natural is good.

THE FACT THAT WE ARE STILL HERE DOES NOT SHOW THAT CHILDBIRTH IS INHERENTLY SAFE

Romanticizing childbirth involves romanticizing evolution. *Natural* is not a synonym for *safe*, and we understand that in other areas of life. For example, tobacco, cocaine, and snake venom are natural; they are not safe. Hurricanes and earthquakes are 100 percent natural, and yet they are responsible for death, suffering, and destruction. Natural means one thing only: it happens in nature. The word tells us absolutely nothing about whether what we are talking about is safe or dangerous.

Many natural childbirth advocates claim that childbirth must be safe because "we are still here." As British midwife Sara Wickham writes:

> [R]emember that women have been having babies
> for millions of years—without the aid of hospitals or
> medical intervention. And if birth didn't work, then
> we wouldn't be here now! Women's bodies are designed
> to have babies. Trust your body. Trust your baby. Trust
> birth.[12]

This claim reflects a fundamental lack of knowledge about
evolution. The fact that "we are still here" tells us only that in
every generation, the number of people who lived exceeded those
who died. It doesn't tell us anything about the ratio. So, for example, the human population will grow at a certain rate if each couple has three surviving children. It does not matter whether the
couple had three children, all of whom survived, or ten children,
seven of whom died.

We know from the biology of other animals that reproduction
has a tremendous amount of wastage. We've all seen documen-
taries about sea turtles that lay hundreds of eggs, yet only a few
baby turtles survive the treacherous clamber across the beach to
the safety of the ocean. We know that some animals, like salmon,
give up their own lives in the process of reproduction. There is a
tremendous amount of wastage in human reproduction, too. The
miscarriage rate for established pregnancies is 20 percent.[13] That
means that one in five pregnancies will not result in a live birth.
Without modern obstetrics, many women and babies did not survive the process of pregnancy and childbirth. These deaths were a
natural part of human reproduction.

In nature, before the advent of modern obstetrics in the early
twentieth century, up to 1 percent of human births resulted in the
death of the mother. To put a 1 percent maternal mortality rate in
perspective, it is twice as high as the mortality rate for receiving

a kidney transplant, and a bit less than half the mortality rate of having triple bypass heart surgery. Despite the inherent dangers to women delivering children, it is eye-opening to realize that the chance of the baby's dying has always been dramatically higher than that of the mother's death. Approximately 7 out of every 100 babies died, compared to approximately 7 per 10,000 today (i.e., a hundred times smaller).

A POSSIBLE DEATH SENTENCE WITH EVERY PREGNANCY

How unfortunate then that contemporary natural childbirth advocates have forgotten the experiences of women who lived before the advent of modern obstetrics. Consider the long history of childbirth prayers.

As Professor Delores LaPratt notes in "Childbirth Prayers in Medieval and Early Modern England,"[14] childbirth was recognized as agonizing long before obstetricians existed:

> *Have mercy upon me, O Lord, have mercy upon me thy sinful servant, and woeful handmaid, who now in my greatest need and distress, do seek thee: behold, with grievous groans & deep sighs, I cry unto thee for mercy.*

As life-threatening to the mother:

> *O My Lord God, I thank thee with all my heart, wit, understanding, and power, for thou hath vouchsafed to deliver me out of this most dangerous travail.*

And as dangerous for the baby, as indicated by this incantation meant to be uttered while stepping over her husband:

Up I go, step over you
with a living child, not a dead one,
with a full-born one, not a doomed one.

LaPratt concludes that these prayers represent the pervasive fear of death and disability as a result of childbirth.

In "Under the Shadow of Maternity: American Women's Responses to Death and Debility Fears in Nineteenth-Century Childbirth,"[15] Judith Walzer Leavitt explores the ways in which the constant fear of death in childbirth, and the frequent experience of the deaths of sisters and friends in childbirth, shaped the lives of women in the nineteenth century. She writes:

> Young women perceived that their bodies, even when healthy and vigorous, could yield up a dead infant or could carry the seeds of their own destruction. . . . Nine months' gestation could mean nine months to prepare for death. A possible death sentence came with every pregnancy.

Natural childbirth advocates appear to be unaware or unwilling to acknowledge the reality of permanent disability due to childbirth:

> For some women, the fears of future debility were more disturbing than fears of death. Vesicovaginal and rectovaginal fistulas . . . which brought incontinence and constant irritation to sufferers; unsutured perineal tears of lesser degree, which may have caused significant daily discomforts; major infections; and general weakness and failure to return to prepregnant physical vigor threatened young women in the prime of life.

Prior to the advent of modern obstetrics, it seems that very few women were empowered by childbirth. The testimony of individual women is heart-rending:

Josephine Preston Peabody wrote in her diary of the "most terrible day of [her] life," when she delivered her firstborn, the "almost inconceivable agony" she lived through during her "day-long battle with a thousand tortures and thunders and ruins." Her second confinement brought "great bodily suffering," and her third, "the nethermost hell of bodily pain and mental blankness. . . . The will to live had been massacred out of me, and I couldn't see why I had to."

"Between oceans of pain," wrote one woman of her third birth in 1885, "there stretched continents of fear; fear of death and dread of suffering beyond bearing." Surviving a childbirth did not allow women to forget its horrors. Lillie M. Jackson, recalling her 1905 confinement, wrote: "While carrying my baby, I was so miserable . . . I went down to death's door to bring my son into the world, and I've never forgotten. Some folks say one forgets, and can have them right over again, but today I've not forgotten, and that baby is 36 years old." Too many women shared with Hallie Nelson her feelings upon her first birth: "I began to look forward to the event with dread, if not actual horror." Even after Nelson's successful birth, she "did not forget those awful hours spent in labor."

That is the reality of premodern-era childbirth, not the airbrushed, made-up fantasy of natural childbirth advocates.

ESPECIALLY DANGEROUS FOR BABIES

Around the world, the day of birth is the single most dangerous day of childhood. As difficult as it may be to read, the fact is that more deaths occur on the day of birth than on any day in the subsequent eighteen years.[16] Modern obstetrics has changed that, but birth has never been and may never be totally safe for babies.

The tragic death of babies is measured in several different ways, and it is very important to understand what statistic is being used. Death can be described as intrapartum (during labor), perinatal (around the time of birth, which includes stillbirths, deaths during labor, deaths immediately following labor, and deaths up to seven to twenty-eight days after birth), or neonatal (from birth to twenty-eight days after birth). This is in contrast to infant mortality, which usually measures deaths up to one year after birth.

Natural childbirth advocates often point to the relatively high (among industrialized countries) US infant mortality rate as an indictment of modern obstetrics. In addition to there being many reasons for the relatively high US infant mortality rate (poverty, race, lack of health insurance), it is important to understand that infant mortality is a measure of *pediatric* care, including as it does sudden infant death syndrome (SIDS), auto accidents, and child abuse. According to the World Health Organization, the best measure of obstetric care is perinatal mortality. WHO data shows that the US perinatal mortality rate is among the lowest in the world.[17]

Modern obstetrics has had the biggest impact on deaths of babies in labor, to the point where infant death in labor is virtually nonexistent in first world countries. When a complication occurs during labor, immediate delivery (usually C-section) can be performed. But obstetrics is more than treating emergencies; it is fundamentally preventive medicine. As everyone knows, it is far better to prevent a complication than to have to treat it. Most of modern obstetrics is devoted to anticipating and preventing complications.

The picture becomes even clearer when one looks at third world countries where there is limited access to modern obstetrics— places like Afghanistan, Mali, and Somalia. Here the mortality rate can be 70 in every 1,000 births, or higher.[18] In other words, 7 percent of all babies (or more) die during labor or in the immediate period thereafter.

The statistics are even more dramatic when you look at the death rates associated with specific complications in third world countries. The perinatal death rate for obstructed labor (a baby too big to fit) is over 60 percent, a staggering figure.[19] Compare that to a death rate of essentially zero for obstructed labor in the United States. The death rate for breech presentation is over 20 percent in some of these developing countries, such as Cameroon[20]— in other words, one out of five babies who started labor in the breech position died—while the death rate due to breech delivery by C-section in the United States is virtually zero. Of the women who developed eclampsia (seizures) during labor in parts of the world where there is little modern obstetrics, 40 percent may lose their babies. Compare that to the United States, where eclampsia is almost unheard of.[21]

Of course, if you believe that childbirth is inherently safe, as many natural childbirth advocates do, the outcome (a healthy baby and a healthy mother) is taken for granted. That leads to a tremendous gulf in outlook between obstetricians and natural childbirth advocates.

Obstetricians are focused on *outcome*. For obstetricians, a successful birth is one where the baby and mother end up healthy, regardless of how that is accomplished. For natural childbirth advocates, who believe a good outcome is virtually guaranteed, the *process* takes central importance. And when it comes to process, for the natural childbirth movement, there is nothing more important than "normal" (unmedicated, vaginal) birth.

NORMAL BIRTH, THE HOLY GRAIL OF NATURAL CHILDBIRTH

If you search for scientific papers about "normal birth" (or physiological birth, as it is also known), you will find very few references prior to 2007, when the expression was popularized by midwifery organizations. The Royal College of Midwives in Britain started their Campaign for Normal Birth,[22] and papers began to appear with titles like "Preserving Normal Birth"[23] and "Normal Birth: Women's Stories."[24]

"Normal birth" arose in response to criticism that midwives referred to unmedicated vaginal birth as "natural," implying that babies born by C-section were somehow unnatural. The real question is: Why did midwives feel the need to segregate unmedicated vaginal birth as somehow different and better than births with pain medication or by C-section?

What does it really mean to call a birth "normal"?

According to the Royal College of Midwives, "Achieving normal births for the majority of women and normalising the process of birth for all women regardless of the type of labour and birth they will experience is our focus."

Why normality?

According to British midwifery professor Soo Downe:

Most women, in every country across the world, would prefer to give birth as physiologically as possible. For most women and babies, this is also the safest way to give birth, and to be born, wherever the birth setting.

Professor Downe is wrong on both counts. When given the choice, most women choose hospitals, interventions, and epidurals. Moreover, there is no evidence of any kind that "physiological" birth is safer than any other form of birth.

It would be more accurate to say that most *midwives* would prefer to attend births that are as physiological as possible. Why?

It is not a coincidence that "normal" birth involves only the things that midwives can do. Anything that only a doctor can do is regarded as an intervention. Some natural childbirth advocates actually debate whether a woman who has a C-section has given birth at all, let alone had a "normal" birth!

Although advocates like to pretend that natural childbirth recapitulates birth in nature, contemporary natural childbirth actually does involve technology. If you were a fly on the wall at a typical natural childbirth, you'd see a midwife checking blood pressure, listening to the fetal heart with a Doppler, or resuscitating a newborn with oxygen. Midwives will also recommend herbs or over-the-counter medications like castor oil to stimulate labor and prevent a term pregnancy from extending into a higher-risk postterm pregnancy. Where the line between "intervention" and "natural" is drawn is fuzzy and arbitrary.

As anthropologist Margaret MacDonald explains in a piece in *The Lancet* entitled "The Cultural Evolution of Natural Birth,"[25] "[If an intervention] can bring back the clinical normalcy of the labour pattern and keep it within the midwifery scope of practice, it is generally regarded as a good thing by midwives and clients alike."

WHO'S WHO IN THE WORLD OF NATURAL CHILDBIRTH

As noted above, natural childbirth is an alternative world of internal legitimacy. It has its own books, journals, conferences, and titles. It also has its own "experts," many of whom are self-proclaimed and most of whom are not recognized as experts except by other natural childbirth advocates.

Grantly Dick-Read and Fernand Lamaze are recognized as the intellectual founders of the natural childbirth movement. Both Dick-Read and Lamaze were older white male physicians. Indeed, one of the fundamental ironies of the natural childbirth movement is that nearly all of its intellectual founders were older white men. These included Frédérick Leboyer, who promoted waterbirth; Robert Bradley, who developed the Bradley Method of "husband-coached" childbirth; Michel Odent, who has provided intellectual cover by fabricating theories on childbirth pain and bonding; and more recently, Marsden Wagner, who during his tenure at the World Health Organization promoted an "optimal" C-section rate that had no basis in fact and was essentially conjured from thin air.

The leading female exponent of the American natural childbirth movement is Ina May Gaskin. Gaskin calls herself a midwife, but she's actually a layperson with no training in obstetrics or nursing. She is credentialed as a certified professional midwife (CPM), a subclass of midwife that exists only in the United States. CPMs do not meet the international standards of education and training of all other midwives in the industrialized world.

Gaskin's base of operations, The Farm, is a cult-like commune founded and led by her second husband, the late Stephen Gaskin, who was revered as a prophet at The Farm. His group restricted women to traditionally female roles, and it fell to his wife to deliver babies. Ina May is recognized as the "grandmother" of American homebirth midwives. She lost one of her own children at homebirth when he was born prematurely, struggled to breathe for twelve hours, and then died.

Most of the other female exponents of natural childbirth in the United States are similarly un- or undertrained. Henci Goer, a self-proclaimed "expert" on obstetric research and author of a shelf of books promoting natural childbirth, including *The Thinking Woman's Guide to a Better Birth*, is a layperson with no midwifery or nursing training at all. She also lacks advanced training in science or statistics. She is not recognized as an expert by anyone outside of the natural childbirth world.

Barbara Harper, the "expert" on waterbirth, is a nurse with no training in newborn physiology. Penny Simkin, who has written extensively on natural childbirth, is a physical therapist. The intellectual leaders of the natural childbirth movement come from many countries, and most are sociologists and anthropologists who lack any medical midwifery or medical training; these include Sheila Kitzinger and Robbie Davis-Floyd, among others.

The bottom line is that contemporary natural childbirth was promulgated by older white men and has been propagated by women who lack even the most basic medical training. It's hardly surprising then that even the most cherished axioms of natural childbirth have no basis in science.

PREGNANCY IS NOT A DISEASE

The phrase "Pregnancy is not a disease" has become one of the most beloved tropes of the natural childbirth movement. Obstetricians don't treat pregnancy as a disease, either. What obstetricians aim to do is assure safety and health through preventive measures and interventions to prevent complications. Here are some examples.

Labor pain is not a disease. Indeed, pain itself is not a disease, just the body's response to a painful stimulus, but that does not mean it isn't worthy of treatment by doctors.

A baby suffocating to death from shoulder dystocia does not have a disease, but is in need of treatment.

Fecal incontinence from a third-degree perineal (vaginal) tear is not a disease, but doctors know how to prevent and treat it.

Postterm pregnancy is not a disease, but it can lead to tragic results.

Postpartum hemorrhage is not a disease, but it kills many women each year, even in first world countries.

Neonatal hypoxia (lack of oxygen to the baby) in labor is not a disease, but it is incredibly dangerous and can permanently injure or even kill babies—and can be treated with supplemental oxygen and/or immediate delivery by C-section.

Claiming that "pregnancy is not a disease" is like claiming that a gunshot is not a disease, and thus you should be allowed to heal unhindered.

In other words, it is nonsense.

TRUST BIRTH?

Another beloved trope of natural childbirth is "trust birth." Carla Hartley of the Trust Birth Initiative explains:

> We stand on the belief that we are born to trust birth; but have been taught not to. Women are obviously designed to give birth and therefore must have been born to Trust Birth. We have been taught that birth is scary and must be left to the experts. *We have been taught a pack of lies.* . . . "Birth is Safe; Interference is Risky!"[26]

But what does trusting birth mean on a practical level?

Simply put, in order to "trust birth," a woman must trust that her baby will fit, that her baby will endure labor, and that her baby will withstand any serious challenges of the transition from life in the uterus to life outside. Most babies do—but not all. That is where medical intervention comes in.

Trusting that the baby will fit may be foolish, but it is usually not dangerous. There are many factors that determine whether a specific baby in a specific position will fit through a specific pelvis. All the "trusting" in the world makes no difference, but enduring many hours of fruitless labor is usually not harmful, and eventually it will become crystal clear that the baby does not fit.

How about trusting placentas? That is really what you are trusting when you "trust" that your baby will handle labor. In large part, trusting birth means trusting the placenta to provide the baby with enough oxygen to tolerate contractions. During contractions, blood flow to the uterus (and therefore to the placenta) is cut off. In this period of time, the baby is, in essence, holding its breath. Most babies tolerate this pretty well because between contractions the placenta provides so much oxygen that the baby has a reserve to draw upon during contractions.

What happens if the placenta is not functioning optimally? In that case, the baby develops fetal distress. Otherwise healthy babies can tolerate a fair amount of fetal distress, but with a malfunctioning placenta, doctors will want to perform a C-section as quickly as possible to save the baby. It's like rescuing a person in the early stages of drowning. If you save someone who can't swim early enough, before they have gone too long without air, he or she will be perfectly fine. C-sections done in the early phase of fetal distress produce healthy, apparently nondistressed babies. But as is true in the case of a drowning person, that doesn't mean they would have survived if you had refused to rescue them.

"Trusting birth" sounds sweetly spiritual; "trusting the placenta," not so much. But that is what you are doing in trusting birth: you are trusting a specific placenta to support a specific baby through a specific labor. You need to be quite confident that you are right; the baby's life is literally depending on it. Because the placenta is an organ, capable of being damaged, diseased, or failing altogether, there is no guarantee your placenta will be able to do its job of providing your baby enough oxygen to tolerate contractions, and until labor happens, there is no way of knowing.

The same thing applies to other aspects of childbirth. Trusting birth means trusting babies to assume a position compatible with safe delivery, trusting your pelvis to be large enough to accommodate the baby, trusting your uterus to contract strongly enough to push the baby through, trusting the umbilical cord not to have a knot in it or not to be wrapped tightly around the baby's neck, and trusting that when the baby is born he or she will easily make the transition to breathing air. Yet complications are both common and natural, subject to purely random forces, and unpredictable before labor begins.

The corollary of trusting birth is "fighting fear" of childbirth. What do natural childbirth advocates mean when they claim they want to fight fear?

Here's what UK midwives Sheena Byrom and Soo Downe say in *The Roar Behind the Silence*[27] in the section entitled "Fear as a Driving Principle of Maternity Care Design and Delivery": "For midwives and obstetricians, fear of recrimination, litigation, negative media exposure and loss of livelihood potentially contributes to defensive practice."

Of course none of these things—recrimination, litigation, negative media exposure, and loss of livelihood—occurs *unless* a baby or mother is harmed or lost in childbirth. As security consultant Gavin de Becker, who wrote the book *The Gift of Fear,*[28] noted: "True fear is a gift. Unwarranted fear is a curse. Learn how to tell the difference."

Fear can be extremely beneficial in helping us to avoid danger, while anxiety, generally related to events that are possible but don't happen often, is harmful and may actually impede our ability to avoid serious consequences. For example, it is protective to fear a stranger who is making threatening gestures, but being anxious that every person you see could potentially attack you keeps you from identifying the rare person who might actually do so.

Fear of loss of life (of the baby or mother) in childbirth has been the impetus for the interventions that have saved, and continue to save, hundreds of thousands each and every year. In contrast, the free-floating anxiety that any interventions such as fetal monitoring, epidurals, or C-sections will interfere with the ability to bond with the baby or may even harm the baby makes it hard to detect fetal distress, which actually can harm the baby.

Midwives who "fight fear" are like an auto manufacturer touting a car that doesn't have seat belts, airbags, or other safety devices:

> It costs less!
> Crashes are rare!
> Seat belts interfere with freedom of movement!
> Seat belts could trap you in the event of a car fire!
> Fight fear of being killed in a car crash!

Most of us are savvy enough to recognize that the auto manufacturer who takes this approach has only its bottom line in mind and is encouraging anxiety over unlikely possible events while simultaneously discouraging the protective fear that saves lives by being prepared for a car crash. Similarly, we should be savvy enough to recognize that midwives have their own control of the patient in mind when they are encouraging anxiety over epidurals, interventions, and C-sections while discouraging the protective fear of death and injury that saves lives.

The bottom line is that we should not trust birth because it has amply demonstrated that it is not trustworthy. We should *respect* birth, just as we respect other powerful natural phenomena like wild animals or major weather events. Both lions and hurricanes are entirely natural, but they are hardly trustworthy, because they can *naturally* cause injury or death. Trusting birth because it's natural is like trusting lions because they are cats. We must recognize that while childbirth often goes quite well without interventions, it has the potential to go terribly wrong, becoming dangerous and even worse at any moment without any warning.

NATURAL CHILDBIRTH AND GUILT

One of the joys of being a practicing obstetrician was that I had the opportunity to save lives on a daily basis. One of the frustrations of obstetrics is that saving lives has become so routine that women do not realize that their lives or their babies' lives were saved.

Prior to the advent of modern obstetrics, every woman knew someone who had lost at least one full-term baby on the day that it was born. Today most of us know very few, if any, women who have lost a full-term, otherwise healthy baby.

If contemporary rates of maternal mortality were still the same as they were in 1900, the number of women who died each year in childbirth would exceed the number of women who die of breast cancer each year, and we consider breast cancer to be a terrible scourge. Now it is extremely rare for a woman to die in childbirth, and those who do die generally had serious medical problems before pregnancy. In places where modern obstetrics is not available, women have a lifetime risk of death in childbirth approaching 1 in 15. In contrast, the maternal death rate in the United States is approximately 15 in 100,000, and the lifetime risk is approximately 1 in 2,500.

Because everyone now expects that every full-term pregnancy will end with a healthy mother and a healthy baby, attention has turned to women's "experience" in labor. The pressure to have a baby "naturally," particularly in many circles of well-intentioned, educated, and affluent women, has become a source of tremendous guilt for women who don't perform in the approved way. The first step toward shedding the guilt of having an epidural or a C-section or any variation from the approved performance is to recognize that while unmedicated vaginal birth is "natural," most of the mothers who have ever existed would have given a great deal to avoid an unmedicated vaginal birth.

There's no reason for you to feel guilty if you didn't give birth "as nature intended," because the likelihood is high that nature intended childbirth to be difficult, painful, and possibly dangerous. Statistics and the historical record make this plain.

That doesn't mean we have to fear birth; it means we ought to respect it. It's not a kitten, it's a lion, and we should always keep that in mind. Just as no amount of trusting a lion will prevent him from mauling you if he is provoked, no amount of trusting birth will prevent childbirth complications. It is only sensible, therefore, to take precautions.

< 2 >

Interventions Are Preventive Medicine

For many years, part of my job was to act as backup for a large midwifery practice. The midwives (CNMs) were well educated and highly trained. I slept in the hospital so that I was always immediately available. The midwives rarely called me, but if they called me, I knew something was terribly wrong.

One night I was awakened at two a.m. by a midwife who was very worried about a dangerous heart-rate pattern developed by the baby of one of her patients. She thought that an emergency C-section might be needed to rescue the baby. I headed to labor and delivery to take a look.

I entered the room, introduced myself to the mother, and immediate saw that the midwife was right. The heart-rate pattern indicated that the baby was potentially seriously deprived of oxygen. I told the mother of my concerns and asked her to put on an oxygen mask to deliver more oxygen to the baby. I was shocked at her response.

"Oh, no," she declared, "I'm not going to do that. I know what you're up to because I read about it in my natural childbirth books. You tell me that the baby is in distress to scare me and ask me to put on the oxygen mask, but that's just the first step. Each intervention will lead to another one, and before I know it, my birth experience will be ruined and I'll be having a C-section, all because you like to operate."

"Actually," I responded, without even thinking, "I like to sleep and that's what I was doing until your midwife called me because she is very concerned. No one would like it better than me if your baby was fine and if you could have a quick vaginal birth. The last thing I want to be doing is operating, and if you put on the oxygen mask, the baby might recover and it won't be necessary."

It was her turn to be startled by my blunt response. She looked at her midwife, who nodded in confirmation, and then put on the oxygen mask. The baby's heart rate stayed dangerously low and we rushed to the operating room, where I performed a C-section that produced a blue baby who perked up immediately when the neonatologist began working on him.

Ultimately everyone was fine, but I was astounded yet again that a mother had actually come to believe that obstetricians recommended interventions in the hope that they would lead to C-sections. Where had she gotten that idea?

THE CASCADE OF INTERVENTIONS

In the world of natural childbirth, one of the most feared effects of the purported medicalization of childbirth is the "cascade of interventions." As discussed above, this refers to the belief that even the most minor interventions lead inexorably to more interventions, ultimately culminating in the most dreaded intervention of them all, a C-section.

For example, your doctor checks your progress in labor and finds that you have been stuck at 7 centimeters dilation for three hours. The doctor recommends Pitocin to strengthen the contractions. The Pitocin makes the contractions stronger, transforming them from barely manageable to excruciating. You ask for an epidural to manage the pain. You continue laboring for four more hours but never get beyond 7 centimeters. Ultimately, the doctor recommends a C-section for "failure to progress." If you hadn't let the doctor do a vaginal exam, no one would have known that you had stopped dilating; you wouldn't have gotten Pitocin or asked for an epidural as a result. Maybe you would have avoided a C-section. It's almost as if the vaginal exam led to a cascade that resulted in a C-section.

Is the cascade of interventions real? In one way it is. If you don't monitor for problems, you won't find any problems, so the inevitable first step in the cascade is monitoring of any kind.

Consider: If you don't take a temperature, you won't find a fever.

For a parent, the diagnosis of an illness often begins by checking a child's temperature (an intervention). If it's considerably elevated, you'll probably take your child to the pediatrician. He or she may look in the child's throat (an intervention), take a throat culture (an intervention) and diagnose strep throat. The pediatrician will prescribe antibiotics (an intervention). The strep throat may be cured, but the child may develop diarrhea as a side effect of the antibiotics.

One way to view this episode is as a cascade of interventions that began by taking your child's temperature. If you had not taken it and discovered the high fever, the rest of the interventions would not have occurred and your child would have avoided drug-induced diarrhea. The other way to look at it is to be grateful you discovered and treated your child's strep throat before she could develop rheumatic fever (a common complication of strep throat prior to antibiotics) and that diarrhea, while unpleasant, is by far the lesser of the two evils.

That example sums up the philosophical difference between obstetricians and natural childbirth advocates on the issue of interventions. Obstetricians will advocate the equivalent of taking a temperature when there is doubt about a child's well-being in utero. Natural childbirth advocates will gnash their teeth over the possibility that a small intervention to assess a baby's well-being will end up with a C-section. In their view, that cascade of interventions should be avoided at nearly any cost.

The goal of natural childbirth advocates is an idealized "normal birth" and that goal is irreparably tarnished by "interventions." Therefore, the more interventions involved in your baby's birth, the greater the guilt you are supposed to feel. Does that make any sense at all? To figure it out, we need to know what natural childbirth advocates mean by interventions, and, in contrast, what interventions are really designed to do.

The definition of interventions can vary among natural childbirth advocates, but as a general matter, anything that requires a doctor to perform or interpret is derided as an intervention, whereas anything a midwife can do (like blood pressure monitoring or listening to the fetal heart rate) is not.

Interventions include C-section and induction of labor, but they also include things that aren't directly related to childbirth, like IV antibiotics to treat women who carry harmful group B streptococcus bacteria, antibiotic eye ointment for the baby, as well as neonatal vitamin K shots and blood testing for genetic diseases.

Natural childbirth advocates also refuse to distinguish between interventions chosen for safety and measures chosen for comfort. Hence, pain relief is labeled an intervention in childbirth, even though it would not be considered an intervention for any other person in any other circumstance. Curiously, certain procedures, like acupuncture, craniosacral therapy, and waterbirth are not viewed as interventions even though they are anything but natural. Moreover, some natural childbirth advocates go so far as to claim that vaginal exams, to check your progress in labor, are an intervention. At the extreme end of the natural childbirth spectrum, Carla Hartley of the Trust Birth Initiative believes that hats[1] (yes, those cute knit newborn caps) are an intervention because, presumably, our Paleolithic ancestors did not use hats.

The underlying premise of the denigration of interventions is that childbirth has an ineffable essence that must not be marred by anything other than what our hunter-gatherer ancestors had available. But childbirth doesn't have an "essence." It is a process, analogous to any other bodily process such as digestion and circulation. No one claims that if you eat with a spoon you ought to feel guilty because you aren't eating "as nature intended." Similarly, if you faint every time you stand up, no one claims that it wouldn't happen if you just "trusted hearts." So why should birth be approached so differently?

OBSTETRICS IS PREVENTIVE MEDICINE

Obstetrics is in large part nothing more than preventive medicine. Almost all interventions are efforts to monitor the mother and baby to prevent life-threatening complications, instead of trying to fix them after they occur. For example, electronic fetal monitoring allows for early diagnosis of fetal distress; induction reduces the risk of stillbirth; IV antibiotics for group B strep prevent neonatal strep infection; antibiotic ointment prevents neonatal infectious blindness; vitamin K prevents hemorrhagic disease of the newborn and associated bleeding into the brain.

The aphorism says, "An ounce of prevention is worth a pound of cure," and most natural childbirth advocates would strongly agree with that aphorism—except, it seems, in the case of childbirth. Natural childbirth advocates are quite comfortable with the idea of watching their weight to prevent the diseases of obesity, checking their blood pressure and cholesterol levels to prevent heart attacks, and limiting alcohol intake to minimize the chance of liver damage. No one says "trust appetites," "trust hearts" or "trust livers." Why? Because we know that they, like all bodily processes, aren't inherently trustworthy.

Natural childbirth advocates have a surprising double standard for preventive medicine. No natural childbirth advocate would ever claim that you should feel guilty for having a mammogram that shows no cancer, but they think you should feel guilty for having an emergency C-section for a baby who turns out to be healthy. No natural childbirth advocate thinks you should feel guilty for choosing pain medication if you break your arm, but they think you ought to feel guilty for choosing an epidural, even though the pain of childbirth is arguably worse than the pain of a broken bone. No natural childbirth advocate would suggest that you ought to feel guilty if you have your teeth cleaned regularly to prevent tooth decay, but they might claim you ought to feel guilty for taking IV antibiotics to prevent your baby from acquiring a fatal group B strep infection in labor.

Is there a difference between preventive medical measures in general and preventive measures in childbirth? There isn't any difference that I and nearly all obstetricians, pediatricians, neonatologists, and anesthesiologists can see. The difference exists only in the minds of natural childbirth advocates. True, all interventions carry risks, but natural childbirth advocates tend to grossly exaggerate the risks of interventions and grossly minimize the risks of refusing them. In the world of natural childbirth, the biggest risk of all is the dreaded "cascade of interventions."

WHY THE ANTIPATHY TO INTERVENTIONS?

Natural childbirth advocates have an explanation for why they oppose interventions. It is comprehensive and internally consistent. Unfortunately, it often doesn't comport with the scientific evidence and relies heavily on outdated sociological claims about the practice of medicine.

The opposition to interventions is so entrenched within the philosophy of natural childbirth that it is actually one of the core principles of the current Lamaze philosophy as detailed in "Care Practice #4: No Routine Interventions" written by Judith Lothian and others and accompanied with an analysis by Henci Goer.[2]

Both Lothian and Goer believe there is no scientific evidence to support the routine use of interventions. That's a rather shocking claim considering that nearly all the research analyzed by Lothian was done by obstetricians themselves. Why would obstetricians, the people legally and ethically responsible for ensuring safe outcomes for women and babies, purportedly ignore their own research? Why, if Lothian, Goer, and other natural childbirth advocates are to be believed, would obstetricians deliberately hurt their own patients?

The question cries out for an answer, and Goer attempts to address it:

One must turn to the social sciences to learn why conventional obstetricians fail to see the harm they do. Medical anthropologist Robbie Davis-Floyd explains that every culture develops rituals around birth designed to reinforce the culture's core values. Our Western culture holds a long-standing belief that women are weak and defective compared with men. Neither their bodies nor their brains can be trusted to function as they should. From this follow two corollaries

Birth is a difficult and dangerous process requiring close monitoring and frequently requiring interventions in order to prevent (or correct) the inevitable problems that will arise should the faulty mechanism be left to its own devices. . . .

Doctors—that is, men (until recently)—must make decisions for childbearing women lest their inferior reasoning powers lead them to choose unwisely for their unborn babies.

In other words, modern obstetrics is nothing but useless "rituals," efforts to prevent complications mean that doctors think that women are inherently defective, and male doctors want to control women.

These are also rather remarkable claims, divorced as they are from reality. Why?

1. As previously stated, childbirth is not inherently safe.
2. Preventive care is used equally for men and for women and does not imply weakness or defectiveness.
3. The majority of obstetricians are women!

Goer also advances an economic argument beloved of natural childbirth advocates:

Logic, science, and common sense, however, have no power to affect belief—and certainly not when that belief justifies the status and incomes of those who hold it.

But as we will see, natural childbirth itself is an industry, and the argument applies equally to natural childbirth professionals. Obstetricians have many sources of income; most are gynecologists, and gynecologic surgery is generally more lucrative than obstetrics. In contrast, midwives, doulas, and other childbirth professionals have only one source of income: natural childbirth. If anything, natural childbirth professionals have a greater economic incentive to ignore the scientific evidence, which, after all, was discovered by obstetricians, not natural childbirth advocates.

Goer concludes with a flourish:

> In the end, motive does not matter. Results matter, and the result here is a system that abuses the women and babies it professes to serve. It denies women their right to make informed decisions about their care, and it fails to provide safe and effective care. Doctors should be held accountable for this. The former violates their ethical obligations; the latter is nothing short of criminal.

Results *do* matter. Modern obstetrics, in association with neonatology and general medicine, have presided over a 90 percent decrease in neonatal mortality and a nearly 99 percent decrease in maternal mortality. It happened *because* of the liberal use of interventions. In contrast, the philosophy of natural childbirth has been responsible for saving zero lives. Doctors are held accountable for their actions. In contrast, most natural childbirth advocates are not. That's why they can criticize obstetrics with impunity and never be called to account for misrepresenting scientific evidence or putting the lives of mothers and babies at risk.

We should ask ourselves which is more likely, that obstetricians are ignoring their own scientific evidence and callously risking the lives they are legally and ethically mandated to protect in order to profit *or* that natural childbirth professionals are ignoring the scientific evidence that obstetricians discovered and refusing to accept any responsibility for outcomes as a result of their own advice in order to profit.

This is just the question we will grapple with in later chapters.

Although natural childbirth advocates oppose nearly all interventions on principle, some interventions are targets of their particular ire: electronic fetal monitoring (EFM), induction of labor, and the use of Pitocin to strengthen uterine contractions. These technological advances have aided in the healthy delivery of millions of babies, and yet natural childbirth advocates recommend girding yourself against them by making a birth plan, even though birth plans have never been shown to improve outcomes and are often simply a source of disappointment and guilt when interventions are necessary.

IS ELECTRONIC FETAL MONITORING USELESS?

Natural childbirth advocates encourage women to believe that electronic fetal monitoring is useless. Consider this quote from Henci Goer, author of *The Thinking Woman's Guide to a Better Birth,* a very popular natural childbirth book:

> Continuous EFM fails to decrease perinatal mortality. . . . Neither does it reduce incidence of cere-

bral palsy. . . . So it turns out more information isn't necessarily better information.[3]

But that's not true. There are two different ways to monitor the baby's heart rate. The first is by listening (auscultation) with a special (Pinard) stethoscope or a Doppler ultrasound monitor. The second method is electronic fetal monitoring (EFM). EFM is Doppler monitoring with two important additions: monitoring the timing of contractions as well as the heart rate to see how the baby responds, and creation of a permanent record, a monitor "strip." EFM can be used continuously throughout labor or intermittently to "check in" on the baby every now and then.

Goer's claim would be more accurate if she noted an important caveat: continuous electronic fetal monitoring does not decrease perinatal mortality *beyond* the decrease achieved by a rigorous schedule of intermittently auscultating (listening) to the fetal heart rate with a Doppler device.[4] That's a standard that is nearly impossible to meet in a modern hospital setting, where a nurse may be caring for two or more laboring women and using a Doppler device according to a rigorous schedule would be too time intensive. That is something altogether different than claiming that continuous electronic fetal monitoring is useless. Moreover, it tells us nothing about how intermittent fetal monitoring (which is typically used for low-risk women in many hospitals) compares with intermittent listening.

Therefore, while we might conclude that it is not necessary for low-risk women to wear an electronic fetal monitor for every single minute of labor, these studies tell us nothing about the value of electronic fetal monitoring itself. The reality is that electronic fetal monitoring (intermittent or continuous) provides much more information than listening to the baby's heart rate.

For example, this tracing shows a baby in serious trouble.[5]

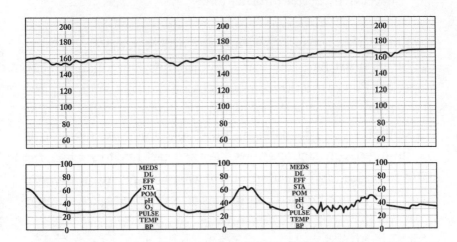

Surprised? You might be if you thought that a fetal heart-rate tracing supplied the same information as intermittent listening. But electronic fetal monitoring provides a wealth of information that cannot be obtained by listening, and that information allows for a more comprehensive view of fetal well-being.[6]

What information does this tracing provide? To understand, you need to know what we are looking at. We are looking at two different graphs created simultaneously by the fetal monitor. The top graph shows the fetal heart rate; the bottom graph shows the uterine contractions. The information in the top graph can be understood only in relation to the information in the bottom graph.

Let's start with the basics:

< **The baseline fetal heart rate is approximately 160 beats per minute.** This is a normal fetal heart rate. Therefore, if you were listening intermittently during the time at which this tracing were created, you would think that the baby was doing fine.

< **There is decreased variability.** We know from looking at millions of tracings that the normal fetal heart rate will create a jagged line. The jaggedness is known as variability. As the blood flow needs of the baby change from moment to moment, the heart rate adjusts from moment to moment. When the baby's brain is deprived of oxygen, the heart rate will lose variability, and the line will look smoother. This heart-rate tracing has lost its variability; this baby is in trouble. There is no way to determine variability while listening, so intermittent auscultation would not alert you to this ominous development.

< **There are no accelerations.** A well-oxygenated baby will move from time to time. That will be reflected in temporary increases in the heart rate (accelerations) lasting for fractions of a minute or more. Without a written tracing, it is difficult to determine if there are accelerations. Doppler heart monitoring does not provide tracings, of course.

< **There are subtle late decelerations.** A deceleration is a brief decrease in heart rate. Their significance is not in how deep they are, but in where they are located in relation to the contraction. They are categorized as early (before a contraction), variable (near the peak of a contraction), or late (starting during a contraction but continuing after the contraction has ended).

The following illustration on page 58 provides a clearer view of a late deceleration.[7] Notice how the decrease in heart rate starts during the contraction and continues after the contraction has ended.

Late decelerations are an indication that the baby is not getting enough oxygen through the placenta to "hold its breath" during a contraction as the supply of oxygen is temporarily cut. Repetitive late decelerations are an unequivocal sign of fetal distress.

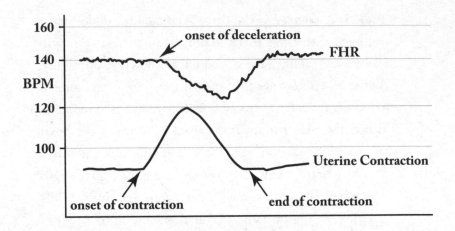

It is important to note that the depth of the deceleration has nothing to do with the severity of oxygen deprivation. Subtle late decelerations, such as those in the tracing at the top, are nonetheless extremely ominous.

Can you hear a late deceleration with intermittent Doppler monitoring? That depends entirely on when you listen, how long you listen, and whether there are contractions during the time when you are listening. The subtle late decelerations in the tracing above might be very difficult to appreciate by listening alone. That's because the heart rate changes by only five to ten beats per minute and for a period of only fifteen to twenty seconds.

Notice what you don't see:

You don't see a bradycardia, a sustained period of abnormally low heart rate. Most babies can tolerate long periods of significant oxygen deprivation before they die, and they may not have any bradycardias until immediately before death. On this tracing, there is never a single moment when the heart rate is outside of the normal range, but the baby is nonetheless suffering from a very serious lack of oxygen.

Henci Goer does not deny any of this. She simply fails to mention it, and it is this failure that is terribly misleading. Intermittent listening is *not* as safe as electronic monitoring. If you can't pick up subtle changes in heart rate, you can't diagnose and treat fetal distress early when the chance of delivering a healthy baby is highest.

Look again at the tracing above and ask yourself, could you (or anyone) hear that heart-rate pattern? If not, then you can understand how very easy it is to listen intermittently to a normal heart rate and then unexpectedly deliver a severely oxygen deprived baby.

INDUCTION OF LABOR

When labor doesn't start on its own and prolonging the pregnancy creates real danger for the mother and the baby, medications can be used to start labor.[8] There are a variety of medications used to soften the cervix and prepare it to dilate, but only one medication that stimulates uterine contractions, Pitocin. Pitocin is an exact copy of oxytocin, the small molecule that causes natural labor.[9]

Why are inductions recommended? A number of medical conditions can pose a risk to a baby, such as diabetes, preeclampsia, and other chronic maternal medical problems such as maternal heart disease that can put the mother at risk too. Anything that can interfere with the flow of oxygen to the baby through the placenta is a potential reason for induction because it raises the risk of stillbirth. It does not mean that the baby will not survive if not delivered within hours or even days, just that the chance of stillbirth is higher

The most common reason for induction of labor is postterm pregnancy, a pregnancy that has gone substantially beyond the normal forty weeks of gestation. That's because, for reasons we don't yet understand, the ability of the placenta to supply adequate oxygen to the baby begins to decline steadily as forty weeks approaches and passes. Not surprisingly, the further beyond forty weeks, the higher the risk.[10]

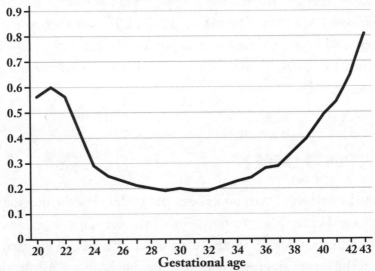

NOTE: The prospective fetal mortality rate is the number of fetal deaths at a given gestational age per 1,000 live births and fetal deaths at that gestational age or greater.

SOURCE: CDC/NCHS, National Vital Statistics System.

For years, the arbitrary cutoff used by obstetricians has been forty-two weeks of pregnancy, because the risk of stillbirth is then double the risk at forty weeks. Recently, however, it has been shown that induction at forty-one weeks actually improves outcomes and does not increase the risk of C-section.[11]

Natural childbirth advocates are certain that induction of labor is usually harmful. According to childbirth educator Judith Lothian:

> Induction rates have increased dramatically. A childbirth educator wonders how she can help pregnant women say "no" to induction. . . . [T]he last days and

weeks of pregnancy as vitally important for both the mother and her baby, insuring the baby's maturity and the mother's readiness for labor. Women are encouraged to appreciate the last days and weeks of pregnancy and to have confidence that when a woman's body and her baby are ready, labor will begin spontaneously.[12]

But the scientific evidence is very clear that induction can be lifesaving for babies at risk because of poor growth, pregnancy complications, and postterm pregnancy. Indeed, from 1992 to 2003, the US induction rate nearly doubled from 14 percent of all pregnancies to 27 percent of all pregnancies. At the same time, the stillbirth rate dropped by 21 percent.[13] Since the primary purpose of labor induction is to prevent stillbirth, the evidence suggests that induction has significant benefits.

Lothian and her natural childbirth colleagues appear to be paying little attention to these facts.

Thinking of, and clinging to, the "due date" as "the day" makes it difficult for women to trust nature's beautiful plan for the end of pregnancy and the start of labor . . . the due date is only a guideline.

That's wrong on two counts. We know that "nature's beautiful plan" apparently includes a 12 percent rate of prematurity,[14] and no one would suggest that prematurity is good for babies. Second, the due date isn't just a "guideline," because the due date tells us how ready the baby is for life outside the uterus. If a woman goes into labor at twenty-eight weeks of pregnancy, no one would reassure her that the due date is only a "guideline" and her baby will immediately thrive.

The natural childbirth literature is filled with stories of women who ignored medical advice to induce labor and their babies survived. That's because induction is recommended when the risk *rises*; doctors don't wait until that risk is 100 percent or even close to 100 percent. The same reasoning applies to putting babies in car seats. We all know plenty of people (maybe even our own mothers) who did not put their babies in car seats on trips to the grocery store, and their babies did not get hurt in car crashes. But the rest of us don't wait until the risk of our baby dying is 100 percent before using a car seat. We want to reduce even small life-threatening risks to our children. Again, what the natural childbirth advocates see as an unnecessary intervention, we see as a preventive measure.

Natural childbirth advocates fear that induction leads to the dreaded "cascade of interventions." That's not what the scientific evidence shows, however. It shows that inducing labor in women who have increased risk of stillbirth actually prevents interventions.[15] That's because waiting renders the baby increasingly compromised, so that even when labor eventually starts on its own, the baby cannot tolerate it and a C-section becomes necessary.

The question for women for whom induction is recommended is how much risk you are willing to accept. Some women are willing to tolerate greater risks to their baby, and some women are unwilling to tolerate any additional risk at all. That's up to the individual woman. One thing is very clear, however: natural childbirth advocates are disingenuous or even untruthful when they advise women that magical thinking ("trusting birth") can prevent complications, that a baby "knows" when to be born (if so, there would be no prematurity), or that refusing induction makes a vaginal delivery more likely. These statements just aren't borne out by the facts.

There is one situation, however, when induction may not be appropriate. "Social inductions," inducing labor for convenience so the baby will be born on a specific day or because you are tired of being pregnant, provide no benefit to the baby and are not medically necessary. But social inductions are entirely different than inductions done for a medical reason and are not what I'm discussing in this book.

There is simply no question that inductions save lives by preventing stillbirth. That doesn't mean that when an induction is recommended, your baby will not survive without it. However, it does mean that your baby is at increased risk, and no amount of trusting birth will change that risk.

SHOULD YOU MAKE A BIRTH PLAN?

Natural childbirth advocates believe that a birth plan is the key to a satisfying, empowering birth. Indeed, birth plans have become so popular that hospitals and obstetricians are offering forms on which women can state their preferences. There's just one problem—birth plans generally don't work. Not only do they fail at their basic purpose, planning a birth, but they often backfire, causing more disappointment than would have occurred without a birth plan.

How do birth plans fail women?

1. **Most birth plans are filled with outdated and irrelevant preferences.** As childbirth educator Tamara Kaufman writes in "Evolution of the Birth Plan":

    > [Women] identify the Internet as the resource they use most frequently to gather information about pregnancy, birth, and birth plans. . . . [M]any of the birth plans detailed on these sites are outdated.

For example, several on-line, interactive tools start with questions regarding being shaved or receiving an enema. Because these procedures are no longer routine in most areas, such details may . . . cause the hospital staff to dismiss the couple as being uneducated regarding routine hospital procedures.[16]

2. **Birth plans are needlessly provocative**, as Kaufman notes:

> On-line birth plans also have a tendency to use phrases such as "unless absolutely or medically necessary"—a phrase that is not always useful when caregivers usually believe the intervention they recommend *is* medically necessary at the time.

3. **Birth plans have no impact on outcomes.** The most important component of any birth plan is pain relief. As Pennell et al point out in "Anesthesia and Analgesia-Related Preferences and Outcomes of Women Who Have Birth Plans":

> Analgesic preferences were reported to be the most important birth plan request. Greater than 50% of women requested to avoid epidural analgesia; however, 65% of women received epidural analgesia. On follow-up, greater than 90% of women who received epidural analgesia reported being pleased.[17]

4. **Birth plans encourage unrealistic expectations.** Just
the idea itself is unrealistic. It's like having a "weather
plan" for your wedding day. There is very little that can
be planned about birth: not the timing, not the length
of labor, not the amount of pain experienced, not the
relative size of the baby's head and the mother's pelvis, not the adequacy of contractions, and not how well
the baby tolerates labor. Yet all birth plans implicitly
assume that labor with fall in the normal range in every
possible parameter. It's not surprising that women are
often disappointed.

In "Is the Childbirth Experience Improved by a Birth Plan?"
Lundgren et al[18] were surprised to find:

> In the birth plan group, women gave significantly lower
> scores for the relationship to the first midwife they met
> during delivery, with respect to listening and paying
> attention to needs and desires, support, guiding, and
> respect.

It appears that the birth plan may have actually set women up
to be disappointed with their birth experience.

The obstetrician's goal is to make sure that mothers' pregnancy complications are treated or prevented and that women give
birth to healthy babies. Unfortunately, many women are so mis-
informed about birth and are so sure (erroneously) that complications are vanishingly rare that they've confused birth with a piece
of performance art. Birth plans are not about birth; they're about
creating the most aesthetically pleasing tableau, one that may not
be realistic or compatible with safety.

By all means share your most important preferences with your providers, but think long and hard before you present your provider with a list of absolute refusals and ultimatums.

WATERBIRTH, AN APPROVED INTERVENTION

Curiously, there is one intervention that is approved despite the fact that there is no evidence that it occurs in nature. That intervention is using a pool of water for pain relief and delivering the baby directly into the pool. No primates give birth in water and no human societies give birth in water with the possible (and possibly apocryphal) exception of a Pacific Coast Native American tribe.

It might seem surprising that natural childbirth advocates promote an intervention for pain when they are thoroughly opposed to epidurals or any other form of pain relief. It's not surprising, though, when you consider that in the natural childbirth cosmology, an intervention is anything that a physician can do that a midwife can't do. Ironically, waterbirth is so beloved of natural childbirth advocates that it is often called "the midwives' epidural."

Midwives introduced waterbirth into their practice without any studies of safety or efficacy having been done. Studies that were performed later have shown that immersion in water can provide some degree of pain relief for some women and there are no risks to the mother or baby from laboring in a pool of water. In contrast, giving birth to the baby in water is actually quite dangerous, since the baby's first breath may be a lungful of water.

The first large-scale look at the safety of waterbirth was a survey that revealed that out of 4,030 babies delivered in water, 34 were admitted to intensive care nurseries. According to the study:

Fifteen of the survivors had lower respiratory tract problems, variously labelled as pneumonia, transient tachypnoea of the newborn, or "wet lung"; suspected aspiration; meconium aspiration; water aspiration; and "freshwater drowning" . . .

[Brain damage due to lack of oxygen] was reported in 5 surviving children . . . including the baby in whom freshwater drowning was diagnosed. . . .

Five babies had a snapped umbilical cord [due to a baby with a short cord being pulled from the water quickly] of whom 1 required a transfusion.[19]

Waterbirth was first mentioned as a treatment for labor pain in nineteenth-century Russia. It became popular in the United States in large part due to the efforts of nurse Barbara Harper. She understood that the biggest risk to babies was inhaling the water from the birth pool, but then crafted four purported reasons why that could not happen: prostaglandins, hypoxia, water tonicity, and the dive reflex.[20]

Let's look at each claim individually.

1. Harper claims prostaglandin E2 causes a slowing down or stopping of the fetal breathing movements.

    That's both untrue and irrelevant. It is untrue because there is not a single study on humans or animals to support it. It's irrelevant because fetal breathing movements (practice breathing in the womb) are not the source of a baby's initial drive to breath. Lack of oxygen and buildup of carbon dioxide stimulate neonatal breathing.

2. Harper insists that the lack of oxygen causes swallowing, not breathing or gasping.

    That's not merely untrue; it's the opposite of what actu-

ally occurs. Hypoxia (lack of oxygen) makes it *more* likely
that an infant will try to breathe underwater, not less.

3. Harper claims that the water in the birth pool is hypertonic and can't pass into the lungs because "lung fluid"
is hypotonic and repels the birth pool water.

In chemistry, the suffix *tonic* refers to the concentration of electrolytes and other dissolved molecules.
Isotonic is the same concentration as cellular fluids;
hypertonic means higher concentration (such as seawater), while hypotonic mean lower concentration (such
as freshwater).

The water in the tub at waterbirth is hypotonic; that
much is true. "Lung fluid" is isotonic, not hypertonic.
The tonicity of a fluid has nothing to do with what can
be mixed with it. Seawater is hypertonic. Fresh water is
hypotonic. According to Harper's theory, you couldn't
add a cup of tap water to the ocean because the seawater
would repel it. That's obviously untrue.

4. Harper believes that the most important inhibitory factor is the dive reflex.

The dive reflex exists, but it is not operating during
waterbirth. The dive reflex is the reason that people
sometimes survive long immersion in icy water. The
extreme cold suppresses breathing and slows down
the heart rate, decreasing the body's need for oxygen.
The dive reflex works in cold water, not warm water,
and of course the water in the birth pool is warm, not
icy cold.

So there is nothing preventing a baby from inhaling a lungful of birth pool water—water that is, by the way, also filled with
dangerous microorganisms.

What's in the water at waterbirth?

A study[21] was done that attempted to answer that question. The authors of this study were aware that the water system itself can harbor bacteria; therefore they tested the water both before and after it was used in the birth pool. The analysis of the water after birth was shocking. Almost all 200 water samples were heavily (as opposed to slightly) contaminated with various infectious bacteria. In the samples taken after the birth, there was a high rate of contamination with coliforms and *E. coli*.

Coliform bacteria come from the gastrointestinal tract. They enter the birth pool with the feces expelled by the mother as she attempts to push out the baby. In other words, the water in the birth pool is no different from toilet water.

Would you completely immerse your head (eyes open, of course) in the fecally contaminated bloody water of a birth pool in the aftermath of a birth? No? Why would you think it is okay to force your baby to do just that?

HOMEBIRTH

Homebirth is the logical end point for those who oppose interventions. There's no better way to avoid interventions than to give birth in a place where they are unavailable. Homebirths provide no electronic fetal monitoring, no IV Pitocin to induce labor or to strengthen contractions, no epidurals, no C-sections, and no neonatologists to perform expert resuscitations. Women who choose homebirth are betting that they and their babies will have no life-threatening complications. If they guess wrong, their babies may die.

And indeed, that's precisely what happens at American homebirths.

While movies like Ricki Lake's *The Business of Being Born* present homebirth to be as safe as hospital birth, all the existing scientific evidence as well as state and national statistics show that planned homebirth with a homebirth midwife dramatically increases the risk of neonatal death three- to ninefold.[22]

Colorado statistics on planned homebirth show a death rate double that of all births[23] (including high-risk and premature births); California has a mortality rate double that of low-risk births[24]; and in 2012, planned homebirths in Oregon with a licensed homebirth midwife had a death rate nine times higher than comparable risk hospital births.[25] The death rate at American homebirth is more than ten times higher than the death rate for sudden infant death syndrome (SIDS).[26]

There are two types of midwives in the United States: certified nurse-midwives (CNM) and certified professional midwives (CPM). Certified nurse-midwives are real midwives with education and training that exceed all other midwives in the world. In contrast, certified professional midwives (CPMs) are not medical professionals at all. Their "credential" was made up by women who would not or could not complete real midwifery training. CPMs lack the education and training required of midwives in all other first world countries. The CPM is not recognized and is not eligible for licensure in any other first world country.

Most women who have the CPM designation haven't attended midwifery school of any kind. They have completed a program of unmonitored "self-study" and paid the fee.

The data from the Midwives Alliance of North America (MANA), the organization that represents homebirth midwives, shows that planned homebirth has a death rate 450 percent higher than comparable risk hospital birth.[27] Homebirth midwives justify their scanty training by portraying themselves as experts in "normal birth." That makes as much sense as a meteorologist who's an "expert in sunny weather."

No one needs an expert in normal birth; if the birth is uncomplicated, a taxi driver can do it, and legions of taxi drivers have done it successfully and for free. The only reason to have a professional birth attendant is to prevent, diagnose, and manage complications. CPMs cannot do that because, by design, they aren't trained to handle life-threatening birth complications.

What about the safety of homebirths in other countries? Midwives in the Netherlands and the UK have far better survival rates than US homebirth midwives. Moreover, homebirth is integrated into the hospital system; midwives can seamlessly transfer their patients to the hospital and care for them there. In the Netherlands, there's even a dedicated transport system. Unfortunately, there are problems with homebirth safety even in those countries. The Netherlands has one of the highest perinatal mortality rates in Western Europe[28] and the homebirth rate has been dropping precipitously (now approximately 27 percent and falling).

Fortunately, homebirth remains a fringe practice in the United States, accounting for approximately 1 percent of births.

INTERVENTIONS AND GUILT

Should you feel guilty about interventions in labor? Only if you feel guilty about regular Pap smears, breast exams, and routine blood pressure checks. All three are forms of preventive medicine, just like birth interventions.

And as for the cascade of interventions? Will one intervention lead to another and ultimately to a C-section? It might, but that's also the nature of preventive medicine. Preventing serious illness and death means that your abnormal Pap smear might require treatment of precancerous cells of the cervix to make sure that you don't develop cervical cancer in the decades ahead. Preventing serious illness and death means that the discovery of a breast lump might lead to a biopsy, only to determine that the lump is benign, but that doesn't mean that we should ignore breast lumps so we can avoid unnecessary biopsies.

Similarly, an intervention in pregnancy or childbirth might lead to further tests and procedures that in retrospect were not necessary, but that doesn't mean the solution is to avoid interventions. Childbirth interventions are like bicycle helmets. Often they are unnecessary; perhaps you've never been in a bicycle accident or your baby delivered by C-section for fetal distress comes out pink and screaming. But just as there is no reason to feel guilty about wearing a bicycle helmet, there's no reason to feel guilty about interventions in childbirth.

They're just preventive medicine, and they lead to happy and healthy babies.

There Is No Benefit to Refusing Pain Relief

S he was in agony and they were arguing about it.

The mother was in active labor, had reached 6 centimeters dilated, and had asked for an epidural despite initially insisting that she didn't want one. The anesthesiologist was at the doorway and the husband was blocking his entrance.

"But, honey," he repeated over and over again, "you made me promise that I wouldn't let you get an epidural under any circumstances."

"Kill him!" she shouted. "Take him out of the way."

The husband reluctantly stepped out of the doorway and the anesthesiologist entered.

Twenty minutes later when the mother was comfortable, she turned to her husband. "I can't believe that you tried to keep the anesthesiologist out of the room," she chastised. "Couldn't you see that I was in agony?"

He tried to defend himself. "But you made me promise that I wouldn't let you get an epidural no matter what."

"I changed my mind," she replied. "The pain was much worse than I ever imagined."

Forever after I told all my patients this story with the caution: "Please, whatever you do, don't make your partner promise to keep you from getting pain relief. That's an unfair responsibility to put on anyone. Leave yourself the option of changing your mind without harming your relationship."

WHY DOES CHILDBIRTH HURT?

Grantly Dick-Read insisted that the pain of childbirth is all in women's heads, as a result of socialization. Well, as any woman who has had a baby would attest, he just made that up. He went even further and claimed that socialization caused women to fear childbirth; fear led to tension, and tension led to pain. He made that up, too.

Contemporary natural childbirth advocates concede that the pain is real, but insist that it brings a variety of benefits, such as the release of hormones necessary for maternal-infant bonding.[1] However, evidence from the studies of childbirth in ancient times suggests that natural childbirth advocates have it exactly backward. The pain of childbirth is not caused by fear and is not needed to trigger a desirable outcome; instead, it may have been vital to prevent maternal and neonatal death, and is now a vestigial response that is no longer necessary.

Before we consider childbirth in the past, it makes sense to think about the role of pain in the human body. Pain is almost always a sign that something is wrong, perhaps seriously wrong.

Indeed, pain is so important to human survival that it can stimulate reflex reactions. Put your hand on a hot object and you will actually begin pulling it away before you consciously feel the pain. There are nerve circuits in the spinal cord that allow you to unconsciously perceive the pain and pull away, skipping the step of consciously noticing the pain so as to save time and limit damage.

When you think about it, there is no instance of pain that is not designed to protect against damage. At the level of the skin, pain tells us what is safe to touch and what is dangerous. At the level of bone, the pain of a broken bone is so great that it forces us to stay immobile, and that probably helps the bone to heal properly. The pain of disease makes people search for ways to diminish the pain and perhaps improves the possibility of survival from the specific problem. So at the most basic level, there is no reason to believe that the pain of labor is "good pain" or beneficial in and of itself. If labor pain is like all other types of human pain, it exists to warn.

Human childbirth has been around for as long as we have been on Earth. For millennia the death rate of both mothers and infants was extraordinarily high. Evolution would certainly have favored strategies that lowered the risk of death. Perhaps labor pain, like all other forms of human pain, existed to warn women to seek assistance or to alert others that a woman needed assistance.

Assistance in childbirth may have lowered neonatal mortality in situations like breech birth (which usually cannot be accomplished without some manipulation of the baby's body) and may have lowered the death rate from postpartum hemorrhage, as massaging a woman's uterus through her lower abdomen after birth helps the uterus to contract and controls bleeding. Assistance in childbirth must be important from an evolutionary perspective because anthropologists report that all human societies have had birth attendants.

As Karen Rosenberg, a paleoanthropologist who studies human birth, and Wenda Trevathan, a biological anthropologist and midwife, wrote in *Scientific American*:

> [W]e suggest that natural selection long ago favored the behavior of seeking assistance during birth because such help compensated for these difficulties. . . . Pain, fear and anxiety more likely drove their desire for companionship and security. . . . [S]uch emotions—also common during illness and injury— . . . led individuals who experienced them to seek the protection of companions, which would have given them a better chance of surviving.[2]

Wouldn't it be ironic for natural childbirth advocates if the role of pain in labor was to alert women to the inherently dangerous nature of childbirth so they would seek assistance? This would also mean that labor pain has outlived its usefulness. Far from being beneficial, labor pain may have only harmful effects for contemporary mothers.

LABOR PAIN EXPLAINED

There are two sources of pain in childbirth, visceral pain and somatic pain.

Visceral pain[3] occurs mainly during the first stage of labor and originates in the internal organs. The pain is usually diffuse and often hard to pinpoint. It's commonly described as deep, dull, aching, squeezing, or sickening. Indeed, visceral pain may be accompanied by nausea and vomiting as well as changes in temperature, blood pressure, and heart rate.

The pain of contractions is visceral pain caused by the efforts of the uterus to push the baby against the cervix to dilate it and then through the vagina. It is exactly the same type of visceral pain as the pain of a gallbladder attack or of passing a kidney stone.

The second type of pain is somatic[4] or parietal pain, which occurs during transition and the second stage of labor and originates in the skin and deeper tissues. This is the type of pain you feel when you cut your skin. Somatic pain feels more localized and intense and is often described as sharp or burning. Somatic pain in childbirth is the result of stretching of the vaginal opening at crowning and birth.

The unalterable bedrock belief of natural childbirth advocacy is that women should embrace childbirth pain because it is "good pain," but scientifically, there is no such thing as good pain. The pain of contractions and the pain of vaginal stretching do not differ in any way from any other kind of pain. It is carried by the same nerves; it is conducted through the action of the same neurotransmitters; it is routed to the same areas in the brain. It is exactly the same as any other kind of pain. It is not more noble or any less painful.

The best way to block both the visceral and the somatic pain of labor is an epidural.

As Tal recalls:

For reasons that I can't really reconstruct, I decided to try for a natural birth. My mother had easy births, and a friend scared me re epidurals and C-sections. After twenty hours of labor, and five of them stuck at 9 centimeters with back labor and excruci-

ating pain, I said, "I need an epidural." The doula convinced me to try just a little harder, because I had gotten so far already. I agreed, and fifteen minutes later I said I can't wait anymore, but at this point my doc was called for an emergency, and I got stuck waiting for another hour. Finally getting the epidural (with a spinal since I was so advanced) was one of the top ten moments of my life.

HOW DOES AN EPIDURAL WORK?

Epidural anesthesia and its close relative spinal anesthesia are techniques in which the nerve roots of the spine are numbed with a local anesthetic.[5] The effect is similar (and the medications are similar) to numbing your mouth with novocaine in preparation for dental work. However, the numbing effect takes place over a much larger area, leaving you without sensation below the waist. Your labor continues, but you don't feel it nearly as much.

Epidural anesthesia is administered through a tiny catheter (tube) placed in your back, overlying your spine. The catheter provides a continuous flow of anesthetic that bathes the nerve roots of your lower body as they leave the spinal cord. Usually, you receive continuous and complete pain relief. Sometimes, however, not every nerve root is reached by the catheter. In that case, you may have a "window," a small area that is not anesthetized. This can be very disconcerting, but it can usually be fixed by repositioning the catheter.

Just as there are risks to using novocaine for dental work, there are risks to an epidural.[6] No doctor would deny this. But the actual risks of an epidural are very low, and most side effects are easily reversed. For example, epidural anesthesia can anesthetize the nerves that control the diameter of blood vessels and thereby regulate blood pressure. After an epidural is administered, you may experience a temporary drop in blood pressure, which may decrease blood flow to the baby. This could result in a temporary drop in the baby's heart rate (bradycardia). The drop in blood pressure can be corrected with extra intravenous fluid or medication, if necessary, and the baby's heart rate will recover.

Spinal anesthesia works on the same principle as epidural anesthesia and was often used in labor before epidurals became available. Because of its distinct characteristics, spinal anesthesia is now considered more appropriate for C-sections and forceps deliveries than for labor.

Spinal anesthesia requires the injection of anesthetic directly into the space surrounding the spinal cord. It is administered in the same way as an epidural, but no catheter is left in place. Because only a onetime dose can be given, the amount of anesthetic injected is relatively large. This results in quick action (five minutes versus fifteen minutes for an epidural) and dense (strong) anesthesia.

The spinal anesthetic almost always affects motor nerves, and therefore muscle power, significantly. Most women lose control over their legs and cannot push effectively after a spinal anesthetic has been given. These qualities present serious disadvantages in labor, but make spinals especially useful during C-sections. They work fast, allowing for major abdominal surgery with no pain. Best of all, the mother is awake and aware throughout the surgery.

An epidural can also diminish muscle control. That's why anesthesiologists often substitute some of the anesthetic in epidurals with opiates. The combination provides effective pain relief but preserves muscle control.

A more significant complication of both epidural and spinal anesthesia is spinal headache.[7] When the membrane surrounding the spinal cord is pierced (accidentally in the case of an epidural and deliberately in the case of a spinal anesthetic), there is an approximately 1 percent chance of developing a severe headache due to leaking of spinal fluid. The headache will go away by itself, or if it lasts for a while, it can be treated with a special injection of the mother's own blood at the original site, sealing the leak; this is known as a blood patch. A spinal headache is not harmful, but it is very unpleasant, so it is something that women should consider before choosing epidural anesthesia.

CHILDBIRTH WOULDN'T HURT IF ONLY . . .

Many natural childbirth advocates subscribe to the "if only" school of pain management.

They believe that you would not experience childbirth as agonizing . . .

> if only you were more knowledgeable about
> childbirth.
> if only you hadn't been socialized to believe that
> labor is painful.
> if only you had eaten right and exercised.
> if only you had hired a doula.
> if only you hadn't had an IV and/or electronic fetal
> monitoring.

To understand why the "if only" school of management is wrong not only in their understanding of pain but also in their claims about what can and cannot "cause" pain, it helps to apply their claims to other forms of pain. Consider gallbladder pain, a classic form of visceral pain that occurs when the gallbladder attempts to squeeze out bile, but cannot do so because the duct is blocked by gallstones. Would a patient in the midst of a gall-bladder "attack" have less pain if only she was more knowledge-able about gallbladder attacks? If she hadn't been socialized to believe that gallbladder attacks are painful? If only she had eaten right and exercised? If only she had better support? If only she hadn't had an IV and/or electronic blood pressure monitoring? The answers, of course, are no, no, no, no, and no.

Why are all the answers no? Because gallbladder pain arises from the contractions of the gallbladder attempting to push out a gallstone, and is transmitted to the spinal nerves and thence to the brain. The pain impulses from a gallbladder attack aren't modified by knowledge, socialization, diet and exercise, nursing support, or the presence of basic medical safety measures. There's no reason to expect that they would be modified by these factors. Similarly, there's no reason to expect that labor pain would be modified by these factors, either.

No woman (or man) should or would feel guilty about suf-fering severe pain during a gallbladder attack, and no woman (or man) should or would feel guilty about treating that pain with pain relievers. Similarly, there's no reason to feel guilty about experiencing or treating severe pain during labor.

How about somatic pain? Consider the pain from a broken bone and ask the same questions. The answers will be no once again and for exactly the same reason. Just as knowledge, social-ization, diet and exercise, nursing support, or the presence of basic medical safety measures would not be expected to modify the pain of a broken bone, they cannot be expected to modify the pain of crowning and birth, either. No one should or would feel guilty about suffering severe pain from a broken bone, and no one should or would feel guilty about treating that pain with pain relievers. Similarly, there's no reason for a woman to feel guilty about experiencing or treating severe somatic pain during birth.

The majority of mothers who give birth around the world every day have no pain relief available to them and must endure unmedicated childbirth. They don't consider themselves empowered by the pain. The glorification of unmedicated childbirth is reserved for those privileged women who have pain relief available to them and therefore can make a choice. The "achievement" for natural childbirth advocates comes in the refusal to have an epidural when it is easily available. But just as the pain of childbirth is no different from any other form of pain, and just as pain relief for childbirth is no different from any other form of pain relief, refusing an epidural in labor is no more an achievement than refusing novocaine for a root canal. In other words, it is no achievement at all.

SEVERE PAIN IS DISEMPOWERING

Many natural childbirth advocates insist that epidurals are disempowering because they limit movement and sensation, yet there are even more women who find them empowering because they eliminate pain.

Dr. JaneMaree Maher at Australia's Monash University offers a very different way of conceptualizing pain and empowerment, one that resonates with most women:

> [W]hen we are in pain, we are not selves who can approximate rationality and control. . . .
>
> So with this approach applied, it can be argued that epidurals, the most effective form of pain relief, give women control over their own bodies and control over their behavior. They allow women to represent them-

selves to others in the way they wish to be seen, instead of forcing them into a "nonrational" space.[8]

While some natural childbirth advocates value the ability to move above all else and therefore consider forgoing an epidural empowering, most women value the ability to control their own bodies and control the way they behave. For them, pain is disempowering because it robs them of the control they value and the ability to articulate other desires.

The bottom line is that there is nothing inherently empowering about pain or pain relief.

Consider Gavriella's story about her desired unmedicated birth of her second child after her first birth with an epidural:

I got my natural birth, and it was supposed to be So. Much. Better. Well, I was sold a bill of goods. The baby had a smoother start to breastfeeding, but that's more likely due to the fact that I had two years of successful breastfeeding experience under my belt. I knew what I was doing. I did initially recover quicker, but that was probably because the labor was so short, and again, prior experience likely had a hand too. But you know what? The pain I endured left me traumatized. Like postpartum depression/post-traumatic stress disorder traumatized. It's "common knowledge" that natural birth means no PPD. Well, with my first, I had just a touch of "baby blues." With this birth, I was hit by horrible, debilitating PPD. He is fifteen months old now, and I'm only just starting to feel normal again.

Here's the kicker: When my PPD got really bad, I contacted a hotline, both for someone to talk to and to find further professional help. The lady I spoke to on the hotline was a midwife. I told her the story and how traumatized I was. She seemed genu-

*inely confused as to how I could have gotten PPD when I had a
natural birth, because it goes so against the narrative. She also
didn't get why I was so upset about my birth experience. It was
a "dream"—quick and completely intervention-free. Interventions are the traumatizing stuff, not unmedicated birth!*

Ultimately, the decision concerning pain relief in labor
depends on what each individual woman values and wishes to
control. Wanting to move in labor is no more or less important
than wanting to be comfortable in labor.

THE BENEFITS AND RISKS OF EPIDURALS

Epidurals have changed labor by making it much less painful and
much less feared than ever before, but natural childbirth advocates insist that the risks outweigh the benefits. The problem is
that many of these purported risks have been shown not to exist.
For example, natural childbirth advocates claim that epidurals
increase the likelihood of C-section, but that's not what the scientific evidence shows. Multiple studies address this issue; they
show that epidurals do not increase the risk of C-section.

A Cochrane review published in 2011 included 38 studies
involving 9658 women.[9] The authors found that epidurals had no
statistically significant impact on the risk of C-section or neonatal
well-being. Epidural anesthesia did increase the risk of having a
vaginal delivery assisted by obstetric vacuum or forceps.

Furthermore, a 2014 Cochrane review of nine randomized
controlled trials involving 15,572 women found that there was no
increase in C-sections, vacuum or forceps delivery rates between
epidurals given early in labor and those given later in labor.[10]

Nonetheless, natural childbirth advocates continue to peddle the falsehood that epidurals increase the C-section rate. Henci Goer, writing for the Lamaze blog *Science and Sensibility* shortly after publication of the 2014 Cochrane review, still insists that "At the very least we cannot assure women with confidence that epidurals don't increase the likelihood of cesarean."[11]

If childbirth pain is good, it inevitably follows that epidurals must be bad. But as we've already seen, the idea that labor pain is beneficial is a fabrication without basis in scientific evidence. Therefore, there is no reason to feel guilty about pain relief in labor.

But what about the side effects? Natural childbirth advocates would have you believe that the epidural poses serious risks to your baby and to you, especially because the drugs will pass directly to your baby once you receive them.

Is it any wonder that women feel guilty about epidurals when they are subjected to this outrageous admonition from Judy Slome Cohain, CNM, a prominent homebirth advocate?

> Two million American women will take an epidural trip this year during childbirth. . . . Similar to street drug pushers, most anesthesiologists in the delivery rooms maintain a low profile, avoid making eye contact and threaten to walk out if they don't get total cooperation. Women get epidurals for one of the main reasons so many women smoked pot in the 1970s—their friends are doing it.[12]

Such a vote of confidence, right? Of course such claims have no basis in reality.

This issue has been studied extensively, and the scientific evidence shows that little if any medication in an epidural passes through to the baby during labor. That's just what we would expect based on an understanding of pharmacology and of placentas.

1. **To get to the baby, a medication needs to get to the mother first.** Specifically, the medication must enter the mother's bloodstream. A medication can enter directly through intravenous administration, but if the medication is injected around the spine, only some of it will find its way to the mother's bloodstream. Epidurals are injected into the epidural space around the spine, and that means that considerably less medication ends up in the mother's bloodstream.

2. **Dose counts.** The effect of a medication depends on the dose. The amount of epidural medication that makes its way into the mother's bloodstream is very small. The amount that crosses the placenta to the baby is smaller still.

3. **The placenta is not a sieve.** Just because something is in the mother's bloodstream does not mean that it easily crosses the placenta or, indeed, crosses the placenta at all.

The bottom line is that what gets to the baby is far smaller than the amount of medication injected into the mother's epidural space. Therefore, if an epidural does not sedate the mother, it certainly won't sedate the baby.

DO EPIDURALS INTERFERE WITH MOTHER-INFANT BONDING?

This is another of the natural childbirth lobby's favorite arguments. Of course there's no scientific evidence to support that claim, nor any reason to think that an epidural could interfere with mother-infant bonding because there is no scientific evidence that labor pain is necessary for bonding. That hasn't stopped

natural childbirth advocates from conjuring a purported mechanism for the claim fabricated by Dr. Michel Odent.[13] Dr. Odent
is a natural childbirth celebrity. Many people are under the mis-
taken impression that he is an obstetrician. In fact he is a general
surgeon who presided over a tiny obstetrical division within the
surgery department at a small hospital. He insists:

> Oxytocin is the hormone of love, and to give birth
> without releasing this complex cocktail of love chemi-
> cals disturbs the first contact between the mother and
> the baby. . . .
> It is this hormone flood that enables a woman to fall
> in love with her newborn and forget the pain of birth.

No, that's not true.

1. There is no evidence that oxytocin is required for
   bonding.
2. There is no evidence that a complex interaction like
   human mother-infant bonding is mediated simply by
   hormones (as any adoptive mother could tell you).
3. If oxytocin was the source of bonding, women who
   received Pitocin would be more bonded to their babies
   than anyone else. Odent and his supporters get around
   this difficulty by claiming that Pitocin is different from
   oxytocin (false; it is chemically identical[14]) or that only
   oxytocin produced within the brain can have an effect
   on the brain (there's no evidence for that, either).

The claim that childbirth pain is required for bonding is,
sadly, an offensive smear. It is almost as if these people are saying
that without pain, women cannot properly love their babies.

DO EPIDURALS AFFECT BREASTFEEDING?

Epidurals do not affect breastfeeding, and there is very little reason to think that they would. That hasn't stopped natural childbirth advocates from insisting that epidurals interfere with breastfeeding because babies are too "sleepy" to nurse after their mothers receive pain relief.[15] A 2014 infographic[16] created and released by Lamaze International states definitively that epidurals lead to "greater difficulties with breastfeeding."

That infographic was created after the writers at the Lamaze blog *Science & Sensibility* acknowledged that, contrary to their fervent belief, there is no evidence that epidurals interfere with breastfeeding[17] by sedating babies. Indeed, the Lamaze blog notes that the studies that purported to find a link between epidural and breastfeeding were small, retrospective, and of low quality. The rest of the literature finds no link between epidural and breastfeeding at all, or draws no conclusion after noting that confounding variables make it impossible to determine whether there is a relationship.[18] What kind of confounding variables? Mothers who deliberately choose unmedicated childbirth are often more committed to exclusive breastfeeding than mothers who choose formula feeding, so any differences in breastfeeding duration between babies of those who had epidurals and those who did not may reflect differences in the mothers, not in the use of medicine for pain.

None of this is the least bit surprising to obstetricians and anesthesiologists. As noted above, when narcotics are injected along with local anesthetics into epidural catheters, only a tiny amount reaches the maternal bloodstream and an even tinier amount crosses the placenta. Epidural narcotics do not sedate mothers; it makes no sense that they would sedate the babies, who receive a far lower concentration. Therefore, it can't be argued that the mothers are too sedated to breastfeed or the babies are too sedated to begin the natural act of suckling.

There is absolutely no evidence that epidurals impact breastfeeding and no physiologic explanation for why they would affect breastfeeding.

CAN CHILDBIRTH BE ORGASMIC?

Natural childbirth advocates are divided between those who claim that childbirth isn't painful if it's done "right" and those who acknowledge the pain but insist that it is beneficial for women. There's a third, smaller group that makes an even more absurd claim: Childbirth isn't merely painless, it's pleasurable. In fact, it's orgasmic!

No, I'm not making that up. Someone else is, and that someone is Debra Pascali Bonaro, who first introduced the claim of orgasmic birth in the early 1990s in her film entitled, not surprisingly, *Orgasmic Birth*.[19]

According to a sympathetic reviewer:

> [The filmmakers] see that birth can be a profoundly sensual, sexual, and spiritual experience; that oxytocin is most likely to flow and increase when women agree to feel their labors—a process that benefits mother and baby in so many ways before and after birth. Most of these women labor in an intimate environment conducive to letting go and surrendering, enabling them to transcend pain (or not to feel their contractions as pain) and, for some, to experience real sexual pleasure.[20]

Really? Really?! Why would a woman have an orgasm during birth? And more to the point, why would she want to do so?

According to alternative health advocate Dr. Christiane Northrup, "When the baby's coming down the birth canal, remember, it's going through the exact same positions as something going in, the penis going into the vagina, to cause an orgasm."[21]

If that "reasoning" were applied to men, getting kicked in the crotch would also result in orgasm, and there are millions of men willing to attest that getting kicked in the scrotum is anything but orgasmic.

Does orgasmic birth really exist? Ina May Gaskin has hinted at orgasmic ("ecstatic") birth in her writings.[22] She says, "One of the best-kept secrets in North American culture is that birth can be ecstatic."

Gaskin's views on the sexual nature of birth are unorthodox, to say the least:

> Don't let the head suddenly explode from the mother's puss. Coach the mother about how much and how hard to push. Support the mother's taint with your hand during rushes. It helps the mother to relax around her puss if you massage her there using a liberal amount of baby oil to lubricate the skin. Sometimes touching her very gently on or around her button (clitoris) will enable her to relax even more. I keep both hands there and busy all the time while crowning . . . doing whatever seems most necessary.[23]

And:

> Sometimes I see that a husband is afraid to touch his wife's tits because of the midwife's presence, so I touch

them, get in there and squeeze them, talk about how nice they are, and make him welcome.

Drawing on Gaskin's view, Pascali Bonaro "revealed" orgasmic birth. Curiously, orgasmic birth has never been described in any other time, place, or culture. Indeed, the only reported claims of orgasmic birth have come from white Western women who are part of the natural childbirth movement.

Orgasmic birth was conjured to serve two purposes. First, it is the logical endpoint of the claims of benefits of natural childbirth. Second, it is yet another weapon in the war of some mothers against other mothers. A says, "I had natural childbirth," and B says, "Oh well, I had *painless* childbirth," and C says, "Ladies, I can top that. I had an ORGASM during childbirth!"

As Danish psychologist Helena Vissing explains in "Triumphing over the Body: Body Fantasies and Their Protective Functions":

> The terror of birth appears to be denied in the concept of Orgasmic Birth. . . . Less ideal birth experiences are acknowledged, but are largely attributed to the cold-hearted world of hospital obstetrics and lack of a caring and sensually attuning atmosphere for the mother. Birth in and of itself is orgasmic in nature, if only the true nature of birth is invited and accommodated for.[24]

There's another reason for the fantasy: competition among mothers. Vissing cites the work of her colleagues that the tendency of women to compare themselves to other mothers reflects "the deeply-needed reassurance mothers are longing for in their struggles with guilt, anxiety, and ambivalence."

In other words, orgasmic birth is a weapon in the ongoing

effort of natural childbirth advocates to pit women against each other in false competition. It is proof of how far some are willing to go in pressuring other women to forgo pain medication in labor: "It won't hurt; you'll actually have an orgasm!"

WHERE DO FEMALE OBSTETRICIANS STAND ON PAIN RELIEF?

The patriarchal medical establishment is often the focus of the natural child movement, but what about the large number of female doctors? Have you noticed that there is a rather important group missing from the anti-epidural brigade? I noticed because I'm in that group: women obstetricians.

Women obstetricians routinely favor high levels of interventions for themselves. They often have C-sections upon request. They choose pain medication and epidurals when they have children of their own.

Why aren't they on board with opposition to epidurals? Let me count the ways.

1. They have personally experienced the pain of labor.
2. They have personally experienced the pain of labor.
3. They have personally experienced the pain of labor.

In addition, they have a wealth of knowledge about childbirth and its dangers. They have more experience and skill in handling childbirth than any midwife, doula, or childbirth educator. They know that most of the natural childbirth claims about epidurals are factually false.

I find it quite ironic that while women with less formal training in science and male doctors with strong ideas about how women should react to pain like Grantly Dick-Read and Michel

Odent prattle on and on about being "educated" about childbirth and interventions, they don't seem to notice that women obstetricians, the people with the *most* education and personal experience of childbirth, are not on board.

Personally, I think that the people who invented the epidural should win the Nobel Prize, the Presidential Medal of Freedom, and an Olympic gold medal. Their contribution to women's well-being has been immeasurable. I had epidurals with two of my four children, and to say I loved them is to grossly understate the case.

Obstetricians are often accused of rushing to intervene with C-sections because they are too worried about the baby's health and well-being. Would it make any sense, then, that female obstetricians would opt for epidurals if they knew there was any danger to their own babies? No, it wouldn't.

Female obstetricians (as well as female pediatricians, neonatologists, and anesthesiologists) choose epidurals for themselves freely, gladly, and with no fears of harm to the baby. That means that you can too, should you wish.

PAIN AND GUILT

Childbirth hurts . . . a lot. The pain is similar to all other forms of severe pain. The pain is not in women's heads and is not the product of civilization or socialization. There is no benefit to the pain for either the mother or the baby. Indeed, there is some bio-anthropological evidence that from an evolutionary standpoint, the pain of childbirth has outlived its usefulness. Its original purpose may have been to prompt women to seek help in labor, help that ultimately may have been lifesaving. Now women do this as a matter of course. We don't need to be prompted by pain to seek help in childbirth.

There are some who would like women to feel guilty and blame themselves for labor pain. Others would like women to feel guilty for using effective pain relief offered by epidurals; these people want women to buy their products or services to ease the pain "naturally" rather than "giving in" and requesting an epidural. To enhance their own misplaced self-esteem, many would like to view forgoing pain relief as an achievement, even though anyone can "achieve" an unmedicated labor and most women who have ever lived have already done so. And the achievement really should be a healthy baby—full stop.

Two important people have nothing to gain from your suffering: your baby and you. Obviously if you are one of the lucky women who don't have much pain in labor, there's no reason to opt for pain relief. However, if you are like most women, who describe labor as the most painful experience of their lives, there's no reason not to opt for an epidural. It won't harm you; it won't hurt your baby; it won't impact breastfeeding; and it has no effect on bonding whatsoever.

Remember, female obstetricians, pediatricians, neonatologists, and anesthesiologists—those who know the most about childbirth, babies, and epidurals—overwhelmingly choose epidurals for pain relief in labor. If we don't feel guilty, why should you?

< 4 >

The Right C-section Rate

I was hired to replace an obstetrician who had taken another job. I inherited all his patients, even those who were in the later stages of pregnancy.

She came in with her husband for her thirty-eight-week appointment and we discussed the fact that she'd had a C-section previously for failure to progress with an eight-pound baby; ultrasound estimates indicated that this baby was considerably bigger.

"I don't want another C-section under any circumstances," she declared. "A C-section is the worst thing that can happen."

I gently suggested that no, a C-section was not the worst thing that could happen; an injured or dead baby was certainly far worse.

"Sure," she said, "but that never happens."

I was not on call when she delivered. The doctor who cared for her called me at home to tell me, always a bad sign.

My colleague explained that the mother had progressed very slowly to fully dilated and then pushed for four hours. In addition, the baby was in an unfavorable position, occiput posterior:

this means that instead of facing his mother's back, as most babies do during birth, he was facing forward. When my colleague explained that it looked like another C-section was necessary, the mother begged for a trial of forceps.

Twenty minutes later the forceps were applied; the baby was rotated and then easily delivered vaginally . . . with a major skull fracture from the forceps. I visited him in the NICU the next day. He was gorgeous, a strapping ten pounds even, and he was brain dead. His parents opted to disconnect life support a few days later and he died in their arms.

C-SECTION, THE ULTIMATE FAILURE

There's probably nothing that engenders more guilt among those immersed in the natural childbirth world than having a C-section.

As Moira explained:

From adolescence, I had been taught that to have a C-section is to have "failed" as a woman. I had been taught that midwives were the only acceptable providers of care because doctors would only want to schedule women for C-sections so that they could get to their golf game or not stay up late. I had been taught that if a C-section was actually medically necessary, it was a terrible tragedy that a mother could recover from only after many years of unhappiness and a homebirth the next time.

The passage of the baby through the vagina is the sine qua non of natural birth. Some natural childbirth advocates claim a C-section doesn't even qualify as a birth. In this way, having a C-section becomes the ultimate failure. Is there any greater form of shame for a new mother than being told you didn't in fact give birth to your own baby?

The script used to demonize C-sections follows a pattern similar to that used to demonize pain relief. Natural childbirth advocates insist that C-sections are virtually never necessary, and that C-sections are responsible for the higher maternal death rates in the United States than in some European countries.

Ani was initially happy with her first birth, a C-section:

> *Then the guilt set in, thanks in large part to the crunchies and wannabe-crunchies in my former circle of friends. "I'm so sorry for your terrible birth experience," they said. "A C-section? You must be so traumatized!" "You're going to use a midwife next time, right?"*
>
> *My terrible birth experience? Trauma? Next time? I was completely happy with my experience, medical care, and easy recovery, until I started hearing it implied over and over that I shouldn't be. I started to think that maybe if I had just toughed it out, listened to another HypnoBirthing CD, been more committed to natural birth, that I wouldn't have gotten that epidural, my dilation wouldn't have arrested, and things would have turned out better. (Even though, as my husband pointed out many times, there is no "better turnout" than a birth in which I was treated with respect, an easy recovery, and a healthy, happy baby.)*

A C-section is a medical procedure typically done to save the life of a baby who may not survive without it, or whose risk of dying during vaginal birth is much higher than the ordinary risks involved in every vaginal birth. Indeed, rather than deserving scorn, C-section mothers deserve our admiration, because in many cases they are willing to face increased risk to *themselves* in order to decrease risk to their babies.

WHAT IS A C-SECTION?

Amid all the negative publicity about the rising rate of cesarean sections, it is easy to lose sight of the fact that it is often a life-saving operation. Literally tens of thousands, and perhaps hundreds of thousands, of babies and mothers are saved *every year* by this procedure. The cesarean section is probably the single most important factor responsible for the dramatically lower rates of maternal and neonatal deaths since the beginning of the twentieth century, and medical advances have made it safer now than ever before.

Cesarean section is the operation in which a baby is delivered through an incision in the mother's abdomen, rather than through her vagina.[1] It is named after Julius Caesar, as legend has it that he was born this way, and colloquially it is known as C-section.

Why are C-sections performed? There are many reasons. The most common reason is cephalopelvic disproportion (CPD), also known as obstructed labor, which is just a technical term for a baby's head that does not fit through the mother's pelvis.[2] This can happen for a variety of reasons, including an unusually large baby, an unusually small pelvis, or an unusual position of the baby, such as occiput posterior presentation (a baby who is "sunny side up" instead of facing his mother's back). CPD is a diagnosis that can be made only during labor. Lack of progress in labor is common to all cases of CPD; that explains why obstetricians often refer to it as "failure to progress." For example, a woman's labor might progress to 8 centimeters dilated and no further. In that case, Pitocin is typically recommended to strengthen the contractions.

If the labor fails to progress further, despite good contractions for at least two hours, it is unlikely that a baby is going to fit.

You might imagine that every labor would automatically progress to 10 centimeters (fully dilated) and that the difficulty would arise during the attempt to push the baby out. However, in some way that we do not yet understand, the uterus senses that the baby cannot fit. Cervical dilation stops several centimeters before full dilation, and no further progress will be made despite many additional hours of labor. Whether progress stops in the active phase (after 5 to 6 centimeters) or during pushing, it is a sign that C-section may be necessary. If the cervix isn't fully dilated, C-section is the only option; if progress stops during pushing, forceps or vacuum extraction may be used to pull the baby out if his head is low enough.

C-sections are usually recommended for breech presentation (baby coming out bottom or feetfirst). Vaginal delivery in the breech position involves much greater risk to the baby than vaginal delivery headfirst.[3] Often an obstetrician will attempt to turn the baby first; this is known as a version. If the version attempt is not successful and the baby is still bottom first or feetfirst, most women, wishing to minimize any risk to the baby, select C-section as the preferred delivery option.

That's because the largest part of a baby is its head. When the head is born first, it is very likely that the rest of the body will follow easily. In contrast, when the head comes last, as happens in breech birth, the head can get trapped in the mother's pelvis, cutting off the blood supply to the baby because the cord is compressed between the pelvis and the baby's body. This can lead to oxygen deprivation and brain damage. Most C-sections done for breech presentation might be considered unnecessary because most vaginal breech births produce healthy babies. Unfortunately, at present we have no way of determining in advance which breech babies will be permanently injured by vaginal delivery, and many women do not want to take the risk.

Another common reason for C-section deliveries, and probably the most controversial, is fetal distress.[4] These C-sections are performed because the obstetrician suspects that the baby is being deprived of oxygen. The diagnosis is usually made by analyzing the fetal heart-rate tracing, as previously discussed, although other factors such as moderate to thick meconium, fetal bowel movement in the amniotic fluid (a sign of oxygen deprivation), can raise suspicion or lend support to the diagnosis. The obstetrician might test a fetal blood sample (taken from the top of the baby's head) for oxygen content to confirm the diagnosis of fetal distress, especially if there is doubt about the meaning of the heart-rate tracing.

Many C-sections done for fetal distress are probably unnecessary, but then a lot of biopsies of breast lumps are also unnecessary in retrospect. Many babies who experience even prolonged oxygen deprivation during labor probably won't sustain permanent brain damage, just as most women who have a breast lump are not diagnosed with breast cancer. Unfortunately, it is very difficult to determine which babies are in danger of suffering irreparable damage. Obviously, no obstetrician wants to wait until the damage is already done; at that point, the diagnosis is easy—but by then it's too late. If fetal distress is strongly suspected, cesarean section should be performed while the baby is still healthy. Yet when that healthy baby is delivered, it is often impossible to determine if the obstetrician acted too quickly or acted prudently to avoid permanent injury.

There are also some fairly uncommon situations in which C-section is always necessary and appropriate. These include placenta previa (when the placenta blocks the cervix; both baby and mother would bleed out without a C-section), abruption (when the placenta begins to detach before the baby is born; the placenta transfers oxygen to the baby, and any compromise reduces its ability to meet the baby's oxygen needs), and cord prolapse (when the umbilical cord falls out before the baby is delivered; outside the mother's body, the cord goes into spasm, cutting off the baby's blood supply). In each of these cases, C-section is undoubtedly a lifesaving procedure.

THE C-SECTION RATE IS NOT A HEALTH CRISIS

Natural childbirth advocates like to portray the current 32 percent C-section rate as a health crisis. The definition of the word "crisis" is a time of intense difficulty, trouble, or danger. Synonyms include emergency, disaster, catastrophe, and calamity. Few credentialed individuals, or everyday people, would portray the American maternity care system as in crisis. Neonatal mortality is at its lowest level ever.[5] We're finally able to successfully care for premature babies a majority of the time. Women who could never get pregnant before, or could not survive pregnancy, are having healthy babies.

So what exactly is the crisis? According to Jennifer Block, author of the book *Pushed: The Painful Truth About Childbirth and Modern Maternity Care*:

> [M]any caesareans are literally medical overkill. Yet some U.S. hospitals are now delivering half of all babies surgically. Across the nation, 1 in 4 low-risk first-time mothers will give birth via caesarean, and if they have more children, 95% will be born by repeat surgery. In many cases, women have no choice in the matter. Though vaginal birth after caesarean is a low-risk event, hundreds of institutions have banned it, and many doc-

tors will no longer attend it because of malpractice lia-
bility.[6]

Despite the purported crisis, neither Block nor anyone else
can point to a single mother who died because of a definitely
unnecessary C-section, let alone the hundreds or thousands of
deaths that the term "crisis" implies. Indeed, though Block and
other natural childbirth advocates insist that there are too many
C-sections, they can't identify in advance which ones will be the
unnecessary ones, and they offer only the most general sugges-
tions for lowering the C-section rate.

Block, like other natural childbirth advocates, chooses to portray the C-section rate as a crisis because that is the best way
to challenge current medical practice. As Paul Wolpe explains
in "The Holistic Heresy: Strategies of Ideological Challenge in
the Medical Profession," "[Critics try] to portray the biomedical
orthodoxy as responsible for the problems confronting organized
medicine . . . and suggest that orthodoxy is ill suited to solve the
developing challenges to care."[7]

For natural childbirth advocates, the "crisis" is the C-section
rate, which is portrayed as unjustified, unaffordable, and injurious.
A secondary crisis is the increase in the rate of maternal mortality,
which is falsely portrayed as rising due to interventions, particularly C-sections. The reality is that any rise in maternal mortality
is due to a variety of factors: increasing maternal age and increased
incidence of chronic maternal diseases such as heart disease and
diabetes. It also reflects socioeconomic factors. The maternal mortality rate is three times higher for women of African descent. In
fact women die for *lack* of access to high-tech interventions, not
because of high-tech interventions.

As Wolpe notes, the critic of medicine "rarely paints its opponent in terms of benign neglect," but rather claims that it is evil. Therefore, the rising C-section rate is never portrayed by natural childbirth advocates as the regrettable but inevitable result of the desire to prevent all possible dangerous outcomes, but instead is characterized as the result of the obstetrician's desire to get rich, to "get home for dinner," or simply to control (read *ruin*) a woman's birth experience.

The critic offers the new philosophy, in this case natural childbirth, sometimes insisting that it isn't really new but a return to "ancient wisdom."

> [Critics] often import foreign, folk, and traditional forms of healing into their practices, [carefully describing] them as wholly compatible with Western medicine, scientifically valid, or historically present in other forms.

Ultimately, in the minds of the critics:

> Promiscuous use of drugs and surgery represent not cures, but substitutes for curative action. They are distributed without thought and without recognition of their power to do harm.

The bottom line is that the current C-section rate is portrayed as a crisis in an effort to promote natural childbirth advocacy, and is not seen for what it is—an effort to minimize neonatal injury and increase the chances of safe delivery.

INCREASED MATERNAL MORTALITY

The natural childbirth literature often states that C-sections increase the risk of maternal death, but that's not what the scientific evidence shows.[8] While it may be true that more women who have C-sections die in childbirth, their deaths are caused not by C-sections but by the factors underlying the need for C-section in the first place.[9] Such factors are known as confounding factors.

It's a phenomenon that we understand well in other situations. If I told you that the death rate of patients in the intensive care unit (ICU) is higher than the death rate in the rest of the hospital, you probably wouldn't be surprised. You wouldn't conclude that the ICU *causes* those deaths or that moving patients out of the ICU onto a regular medical floor would save their lives. You would understand that it was the disease or accident that made intensive care necessary in the first place (the confounding factor) that caused the death, not the location within the hospital.

The issue of confounding factors is extremely important and is the reason for one of the basic principles of statistics: correlation is not causation. Simply put, just because one phenomenon is associated with another does not mean that the first caused the second. There's no question that higher death rates are associated with staying in the intensive care unit, but the higher death rates aren't *caused* by staying in the intensive care unit.

In fact, if you look at the leading causes of maternal mortality in the United States, most are associated with too *few* medical interventions, not too many.[10] The leading causes include maternal cardiac disease, pregnancy complications like preeclampsia, and childbirth complications such as hemorrhage. In these cases, because of life-threatening pregnancy complications or life-threatening preexisting medical conditions, C-section is often the best chance to save the life of the mother, not the cause of her death.

MOTHER-INFANT BONDING

Again we hear from Dr. Michel Odent. This time he claims:

> What we can say for sure is that when a woman gives birth with a pre-labour Caesarean section she does not release this flow of love hormones, so she is a different woman than if she had given birth naturally and the first contact between mother and baby is different.[11]

As we said in chapter 3, there's no scientific evidence to support his claims and copious evidence to contradict it.

- There is no evidence that oxytocin is required for bonding.
- There is no evidence that a complex physical and psychological interaction like maternal-infant bonding is mediated simply by hormones.
- If oxytocin was the source of bonding, women who received Pitocin would be more bonded to their babies than anyone else. Odent and his supporters get around this annoying difficulty by claiming that Pitocin is different from oxytocin when it is an exact copy, and by arguing that only the oxytocin produced within the brain can have an effect. None of this is true.

This claim is just another effort to denigrate women who have C-sections.

THE "RIGHT" C-SECTION RATE?

Everyone is sure that the C-section rate is too high, and it may very well be that we can lower the C-section rate without raising perinatal mortality rates. Many natural childbirth advocates cite an old "optimal" C-section rate of 10 to 15 percent issued by the World Health Organization (WHO) nearly thirty years ago.[12] They don't realize that the recommendation was quietly withdrawn in 2009, with WHO acknowledging that there were *never* any data to support a rate that low.[13] Indeed there was never *any* research that established an optimal rate at all.

According to the 2009 WHO publication:

> Although the WHO has recommended since 1985 that the rate not exceed 10–15 per cent, there is no empirical evidence for an optimum percentage . . . the optimum rate is unknown.

So who was responsible for issuing an optimal C-section rate that was apparently conjured from thin air?

Dr. Marsden Wagner, a pediatric epidemiologist and a WHO executive at the time the recommendation was issued, probably did more than anyone to promote the idea of a 15 percent C-section rate as ideal. Yet in a 2007 journal article, he explicitly acknowledged that the 15 percent C-section rate recommendation of 1985 was made without any data to support it, noting that his later article "is actually the first paper that attempts to compare international C-section rates with maternal and neonatal mortality."

> Since publication of the WHO consensus statement in 1985, debate regarding desirable levels of CS has continued; nevertheless, this paper represents the first

attempt to provide a global and regional comparative analysis of national rates of caesarean delivery and their ecological correlation with other indicators of reproductive health.[14]

What did Dr. Wagner find when he actually looked into the impact of C-section rates on maternal and neonatal mortality? He found that there are only two countries in the world that have C-section rates of less than 15 percent *and* low rates of maternal and neonatal mortality. Those countries are Croatia (14 percent) and Kuwait (12 percent). Neither country is noted for the accuracy of its health statistics. In contrast, *every* other country in the world with a C-section rate of less than 15 percent has unacceptably high levels of maternal and neonatal mortality.

Wagner's efforts to promote a C-section rate of 10 to 15 percent are belied by his own data. Virtually none of the countries with low rates of maternal and neonatal mortality have a C-section rate of 15 percent or below, and most have rates that are far higher. The data actually show that a C-section rate of 15 percent is unacceptably low, and that the average should be at least 22 percent, with rates as high as 36 percent yielding low levels of maternal and neonatal mortality.

The current US rate of 32 percent is well within that range. Could the C-section rate be safely lowered? That is definitely a possibility. Could it be safely lowered to 10 to 15 percent? Absolutely not.

LOWERING THE C-SECTION RATE

Are some C-sections unnecessary? Almost certainly—in retrospect. The question we face is how to determine which C-sections are unnecessary before safely delivering the baby by C-section. That's hard to do. So it's worth reviewing how we got to a 32 percent C-section rate.

Old movies sometimes contain scenes in which a doctor approaches a father waiting for his wife to deliver their baby. There's a problem and they now face a choice. Should they save the mother or the baby? There was a time when that portrayal was realistic because C-sections were exceedingly dangerous due to the risks of general anesthesia, infection, and bleeding. Since the advent of regional anesthesia (epidurals and spinals), antibiotics, and blood transfusions, C-sections have become dramatically safer. Now we don't have to choose between mother and child; a C-section can easily save both parties. Therefore, the decision to perform a C-section usually depends on the risk to the baby.

As C-sections have become safer, the risks to the baby that we are willing to tolerate have become smaller. For example, at this point is makes sense to perform C-sections for breech babies even though the risk of death of the baby is relatively low.

In addition, we have developed a variety of technologies to determine if a baby faces increased risk. From electronic fetal monitoring to ultrasound examination to testing for gestational diabetes, we can recognize a possible cause for concern. Unfortunately, many of these technologies are imperfect. Although they have low false negative rates (if they indicate that a baby is fine, the baby is almost certainly fine), they have high false positive rates. That means that if a baby is identified as being at risk, it isn't necessarily at risk.

The solution that natural childbirth advocates offer to this dilemma is to jettison the technology altogether. But as previously stated, if you don't take a temperature, you won't find a fever. This is a foolhardy way to approach the problem. The real solution is to develop more accurate technology that produces a lower false positive rate. Then we will have a better way of knowing which C-sections are absolutely necessary, and thus bring down our rate.

C-SECTIONS CHANGE NEWBORN DNA?

It seems there's no limit to what natural childbirth advocates will do to demonize medical intervention. That includes grasping on to and misrepresenting the latest scientific discoveries, such as epigenetics. Perhaps the most laughable claim put forward by natural childbirth advocates is that somehow C-sections alter the DNA of newborn babies.

What is epigenetics, and is there any reason to believe that newborn DNA is changed by C-section?

Epigenetics studies various chemical modifications of DNA that are the result of environmental influences.[15] There are no changes to the genes themselves, but molecules around the genes that switch them on and off are changed. For example, long after a famine in Sweden in the late 1800s, researchers found that the children and grandchildren of people who had survived famine were more likely to be obese than the rest of the population.[16] The theory is that the proteins surrounding the genes that cause the body to conserve calories switched on in the grandparent and remained on in subsequent generations despite the fact that his or her descendants were not exposed to famine. Hence, obesity was far more common in descendants than would be expected if dictated only by the current environment and inherited genes of the population.

So how does this apply to C-sections? It doesn't. There have been preliminary studies that claim to show a difference between the DNA of babies born vaginally and babies born by C-section, but they are small and equivocal, and it is unclear if they have any significance at all.[17]

But that doesn't stop natural childbirth advocates from enthusiastically embracing them. British midwife Soo Downe, who has neither training in nor understanding of epigenetics, has latched on to the research around this to demonize C-sections:

> Getting childbirth right is profoundly important for the wellbeing of families, and for future generations. While I have always believed this intuitively, recent exciting evidence from epigenetics seems to suggest that there is biological evidence for the impact of labour and birth on the way genes might be expressed for the child, and for their adulthood, and then their own children in the future.[18]

In an interview with Scienceline, Hannah Dahlen, an Australian midwife, inadvertently revealed the midwives' primary motivation.[19] Speaking about herself and her colleagues, she noted that they are frustrated:

> [D]espite the research, political activism and efforts [we] and many others were putting in to increase the rate of normal birth, intervention during childbirth kept rising and arguments about safety and outcomes all had a short-term focus [i.e., whether the baby survives uninjured].

Dahlen believes that focus on epigenetics could increase respect and demand for vaginal birth.

What do scientists in the field of epigenetics have to say about the midwives' theory that C-sections alter newborn DNA? They dismiss out of hand the idea that the method of birth has any epigenetic impact.[20]

Louis Muglia, the codirector of the Center for Prevention of Preterm Birth at Cincinnati Children's Hospital Medical Center, points out that birth is a relatively short event and that "you wouldn't want the body to be reprogramming itself every time an event came up. . . . [I]t's a little counterintuitive that the labor process would have as big an impact on epigenetic programming as pregnancy."

In other words, in addition to the fact that there is no data to support a claim that C-section alters newborn DNA, there is no reason to believe that it would. Changing a baby's epigenetic makeup requires events of long standing, and birth is simply too short to have any lasting effect.

BIRTH AND THE MICROBIOME

The 2014 documentary film *Microbirth* [21] was conceived, produced, and funded by natural childbirth advocates in the latest desperate attempt to demonize C-sections. Its fundamental claim is that C-sections interfere with a newborn's microbiome.

What exactly is the microbiome? According to the American Society for Microbiology:

> The human microbiome, the collection of trillions of microbes living in and on the human body, is not random. . . . The bacteria in the infant intestine digestive system is known as the neonatal gut microbiome. The neonatal gut microbiome is known to aid in digestion but some scientists believe that the gut microbiome may play a role in the development of disease.[22]

Research shows that the microbiome of babies born by C-section differs from the microbiome of babies born vaginally. Presumably the difference is that babies born vaginally are exposed to the bacteria of the mother's vagina. No one knows what the difference means; no one knows if one set of bacteria is better than another. No one knows whether the neonatal microbiome has an impact on health or disease. Nonetheless, natural childbirth advocates have begun recommending "seeding" the microbiome of C-section babies by swabbing their mouths with their mother's vaginal secretions.

According to the producers of *Microbirth*:

> We believe "seeding of the baby's microbiome" should be on every birth plan . . . [T]his could make a massive difference to the baby's health for the rest of its life. Consequently, we believe that *Microbirth* is of extreme importance for global health and potentially, for the future of mankind!

Let's leave aside the breathless hyperbole for the moment and ask some simple questions. Who is the "we" when the producers of *Microbirth* announce that "we believe"? It's not microbiologists, since there is no *scientific* consensus on the composition of the neonatal microbiome, let alone what it ought to be. Microbiologists do not yet understand how much of the tremendous variation from individual to individual reflects anything other than the fact that individuals differ in a myriad number of ways. Nor do microbiologists at this point have any idea of the short-term impact of the neonatal microbiome on a person's well-being, let alone the long-term impact. Microbiologists also do not yet understand how the microvirome (the viruses that normally live inside human beings) impacts the microbiome.

The "we" mentioned above are not neonatologists and pediatricians, since they aren't going to believe anything about the microbiome that isn't established by microbiologists. That goes for obstetricians too. So the only people who "believe" that the neonatal microbiome is crucial to the development of the health and future well-being of infants are natural childbirth advocates committed to unmedicated vaginal birth and strongly opposed to C-sections.

VAGINAL BIRTH AFTER A PREVIOUS C-SECTION (VBAC)

Several decades ago obstetricians believed "once a C-section, always a C-section." That's because the type of incision that was used to enter the uterus, a vertical incision, was at high risk of rupturing when the uterus contracted in a subsequent labor. Over time, the preferred method of entering the uterus to deliver a baby changed to a low transverse (horizontal incision). Research showed that once they are healed, transverse incisions are much stronger than vertical incisions.[23] Therefore, attempting a vaginal birth after C-section became far less risky.

Overall, the success rate of attempted vaginal birth after C-section is approximately 76 percent.[24] In the early 1990s doctors encouraged VBACs, and the majority of women who attempted them were spared a subsequent C-section. The risk of rupture of a transverse incision, while greatly diminished compared to a vertical incision, is not zero.[25] Uterine ruptures can and do happen when women attempt vaginal birth after C-section, and babies die as a result. The mother's life is also put at risk by a rupture, and some women must have immediate hysterectomies in the wake of such an event in order to prevent bleeding to death.

Because of these tragedies and the lawsuits they engendered, the American College of Obstetricians and Gynecologists issued recommendations to make attempted VBAC as safe as possible. Since time is of the essence when a uterus ruptures, ACOG recommended that an obstetrician be standing by any time a woman attempted a VBAC. In addition, ACOG recommended that an anesthesiologist remain within the hospital for the entire duration of labor so an immediate C-section could be done in the event of a rupture.[26]

This placed small community hospitals in a bind. While large hospitals always have obstetricians and anesthesiologists available in the hospital, smaller institutions do not. Obstetricians come in when they have a patient in labor, but anesthesiologists often are on call from home, meaning that they are not immediately available in an emergency. It costs a great deal of money to have anesthesiologists remain in the hospital. Rather than spend the money, these hospitals stopped offering VBAC as an option.

Malpractice insurers also took note of the risk of uterine rupture. They reasoned that they would not have to pay for such injuries and deaths if they refused to cover these procedures. Many obstetricians and hospitals now carry malpractice policies that specifically forbid VBACs.

In many areas, particularly rural, attempting a VBAC is no longer an option. Natural childbirth advocates are incensed by the fact that VBACs are no longer widely available and have formed organizations such as ICAN (International Cesarean Awareness Network) to convince women to demand VBACs. ICAN refers to current hospital policies as VBAC bans,[27] but it is important to understand that no doctors have banned VBAC. Either hospitals or insurers have made it impossible for obstetricians to give patients the option to choose the slightly higher risk of VBAC.

WHAT SHOULD WE DO ABOUT VBACS?

Women who live near large hospitals usually can have a VBAC, and the majority of attempts are successful. However, patients who live near small community hospitals and the obstetricians who work in those hospitals are deeply unhappy over the loss of the VBAC option. Moreover, the C-section rate and the downstream complications of C-sections—the need for future C-sections, the risk of uterine rupture in future vaginal births, and the increased risk of problems with the placenta in subsequent pregnancies— have both risen in response.

On the face of it, this is a simple problem to solve: simply go back to allowing every woman who wants to attempt a VBAC to do so. If this was simply a matter of the will of the patients and doctors, we could do that. However, the situation is controlled by hospitals and malpractice insurers, who view the VBAC option as expensive to offer and conducive to lawsuits. It seems to me that instituting more rigorous criteria for attempting a VBAC could lower the risk of complications and thereby make it reasonable for hospitals that do not have twenty-four-hour in-hospital anesthesia coverage to offer VBACs.

NOT ALL VBACS ARE CREATED EQUAL

Natural childbirth advocates are so anxious to promote VBACs that they have lost sight of the fact (and fail to inform women of the fact) that not all VBACs are created equal. Although 76 percent of women attempting VBAC will be successful, that does not mean that each individual woman has a 76 percent chance of success. Both the chance of having a successful VBAC and the chance of a uterine rupture are modified by the woman's past medical history and issues in the current pregnancy.

For example:

History of a previous vaginal birth impacts the chances of successful VBAC. Women who have had a previous vaginal delivery in addition to previous C-section have an 86 percent chance of successful VBAC, and women who have had a successful VBAC in a previous pregnancy have a nearly 90 percent chance of having another. But for women who have never had a vaginal birth, the chance of successful VBAC is only 61 percent.[28]

The reason for a previous C-section also affects the success rate of attempted VBAC. If the previous C-section was done for a nonrecurring condition like breech, the chances of a successful VBAC are higher than for women whose previous C-section was performed for cephalopelvic disproportion, or because the baby's head was too large to fit through the woman's pelvis.[29]

The larger the baby, the lower the chance of successful VBAC. Although macrosomia (a baby larger than 8¾ pounds) in the absence of other risk factors is not an indication for repeat C-section, the size of the baby definitely affects the chance of success. For example, while a woman who had a previous C-section and no vaginal deliveries has an overall chance of successful VBAC in the range of 60+ percent, the chance of success drops to 38 percent if the baby is over 9¾ pounds.[30] And if the previous C-section was done because the baby didn't fit, the chance of a successful VBAC with a baby over 9¾ pounds is only 29 percent.

Other factors play a role in success and have to be taken into account. For example, if the baby's head has not descended into the pelvis at the start of labor, the chance of successful VBAC drops to only 10 percent.[31] Maternal factors play a role too. The chance of successful VBAC drops as maternal age increases and as maternal BMI (body mass index) increases. Women over age thirty-five and women with a BMI greater than 30 have a lower chance of successful VBAC.[32]

The most dreaded complication of attempting a VBAC is rupture of the uterus. The risk of rupture rises as the chance of a successful VBAC declines, whether that is due to circumstances surrounding the previous C-section or the characteristics of mother and baby.

The worst situation for both mother and baby is a failed attempt at VBAC. While the overall risk of uterine rupture is 7/1000, that risk jumps to 23/1000 in a failed attempt.[33] Therefore, the risk of rupture is directly dependent on the chance of success.

Additional factors include the type of incision on the uterus (transverse is safer than vertical), the length of time since the last pregnancy (an interpregnancy interval of less than six months triples the risk of rupture), and the timing of the previous C-section (a preterm C-section has a higher risk of rupture in a subsequent pregnancy than a term C-section).[34, 35]

Should an individual woman try for a VBAC? Natural childbirth advocates think that just about every woman is a good candidate for an attempt at VBAC, but that's not true. *Overall, elective repeat C-section is safer for the baby, and vaginal delivery is safer for the mother,* but those risks are not equal. The risk of death of the baby in attempted VBAC is 10 times higher than the risk of death of the mother from a repeat C-section.

Each woman must decide for herself which risks she is willing to take for herself and for her child, but she can make an informed decision only if she has all the facts. Only a personalized risk assessment, based on her history, her medical conditions, and the size and position of her baby, will allow her to make an informed choice for VBAC or an elective repeat C-section. And that choice is hers alone.

AN ODE TO C-SECTION MOTHERS

In the world of natural childbirth, there is no greater put-down than the accusation that a woman did not have an unmedicated vaginal delivery. That makes sense if you view birth as a completely safe process whose goal is to perfectly replicate life in prehistoric times. However, if your goal is doing whatever is best for your baby, there may be nothing more natural than a C-section.

C-section represents a transfer of risk. Vaginal delivery poses a much greater risk to the baby than to the mother (approximately 100 times higher). C-section, on the other hand, poses a marginally greater risk to the mother and dramatically reduces risk to the baby. What could be more natural than a loving mother opting to carry any increased risk rather than putting it on the baby?

That's why there is never any need to feel guilty about having a C-section.

Actress Kate Winslet was actually so embarrassed about having a C-section for her first child that she led the world to believe that it never happened:

> When she celebrated the birth of her first baby, she hailed the joys of natural childbirth.
>
> But now, four years on, Kate Winslet has admitted she lied—her daughter Mia was delivered by emergency Caesarean section. . . .
>
> "I just said that I had a natural birth because I was so completely traumatised by the fact that I hadn't given birth. I felt like a complete failure."[36]

The feeling of failure associated with C-section is something I've never understood. Personally, I think C-section mothers should be extra proud of themselves. When offered the choice between risk to their unborn baby and risk to themselves, they chose taking on the risk in an effort to protect the baby. If that isn't the essence of motherhood, I don't know what is.

Consider C-section for breech birth. As doctors, we are obligated to tell women that a breech vaginal delivery greatly increases the risk of death or serious disability.

Make no mistake, the absolute risk that the baby will not survive a vaginal breech birth is small, less than 1 percent, but to me that makes it all the more remarkable that most women carrying breech babies will choose C-section. Faced with the small but real risk to their babies, most mothers will opt for abdominal surgery, with all the pain, the potentially harder recovery, and the increased risk of infection or bleeding. In other words, women who choose C-section for breech want to protect their babies from any risk, no matter how small, at the cost of pain and potential suffering to themselves.

The same thing goes for women who consent to C-section for fetal distress. In 2016, the diagnosis of fetal distress is imperfect at best. We know that almost all babies who experience lack of oxygen during labor will give evidence of that on electronic fetal monitoring. However, many babies who appear to be in distress may actually be fine. When a woman consents to a C-section for fetal distress, she is saying in essence: I don't know whether my baby is truly experiencing oxygen deprivation, but I don't want to take any chances. Cut me and help the baby; if I'm wrong, it's a price I'm willing to pay to be sure that my baby is okay.

In other words, it's a sign of devotion, not a sign of failure.

Kate Winslet is not alone in her feelings of embarrassment and guilt, but there is absolutely no reason why she or any other mother should ever feel guilty about having a C-section.

As a mother of four children, I say "Bravo!" I never had to face the choice that many C-section mothers do, but I hope that I would have reacted as selflessly as they do.

Can we have a round of applause for C-section mothers? They certainly deserve it!

< 5 >

Breast Is *Not* Always Best

S he called early on a summer evening and she was sobbing. One of my colleagues had delivered her baby daughter two weeks before and she was having trouble with breastfeeding. I could hear her baby crying in the background.

She had taken her baby to the pediatrician for a weight check earlier in the day. The baby had gained only a few ounces since her birth and the pediatrician was insistent that the baby was very dehydrated and needed formula. He husband was begging her to let him give the baby a bottle, but she wanted to talk to a different doctor first. Perhaps I could tell her how to make enough milk for her baby.

She detailed her efforts. She had been nursing her baby every two to three hours since birth. She had enlisted a private lactation consultant, who had helped her obtain a breast pump and told her to pump in between feedings to "increase her supply." She pumped less than an ounce at a time and the lactation consultant had given her supplemental nursing system (SNS) to deliver the milk to the baby. It involved a thin tube taped to her breast near the nipple so the baby could draw the additional milk while nursing.

The baby couldn't sleep for more than an hour at a time, and the mother was getting even less sleep because of the pumping and cleaning of the pump and the SNS system. In addition to her husband, her mother and her mother-in-law were begging her to feed the baby formula. "But," she told me, "breast is best and I want to give my baby the best." She believed that feeding the baby formula would mean that she was a failure as a mother because she couldn't do the most important thing that the baby needed her to do. Did I have any advice for how she might avoid giving her baby formula?

As it happened, I was still nursing my fourth baby at the time. I mentioned that to demonstrate that I was an enthusiastic proponent of breastfeeding but that it was more important to feed the baby than to feed the baby breast milk. Yes, breast milk offers benefits to babies, but they pale into insignificance when compared with the risks of dehydration and malnutrition. Her pediatrician had been correct when he advised her that the next step for her baby would be hospitalization and IV hydration to prevent seizures and other serious consequences. I encouraged her to focus on avoiding pain for her daughter by feeding her formula, not merely to prevent the discomfort of hospitalization and IVs, but to treat her daughter's gnawing hunger.

"You have done everything you could to give your daughter breast milk, and should be proud of your efforts," I counseled, "but your baby needs *enough* milk much more than she needs breast milk."

I emphasized that there was no reason for her to feel guilty. "Were you breastfed?" I asked. No, she hadn't been, and she acknowledged that she had turned out fine. So why was she worried about supplementing her daughter's feeding with formula?

"It's because the lactation consultant told me that even one bottle of formula would harm my baby for life," she replied.

I was incredulous. Where had a lactation consultant gotten that idea, and why was she encouraging a mother to let her baby starve rather than supplement with formula? Something was seriously amiss.

BREASTFEEDING ACTIVISTS TOUT BENEFITS FOR BREASTFEEDING

Lactivists wax rhapsodic about the benefits of breastfeeding, referring to it as nothing less than the "elixir of life." Here's a paean from the La Leche League:

> Breastfeeding has been shown to be protective against many illnesses, including painful ear infections, upper and lower respiratory ailments, allergies, intestinal disorders, colds, viruses, staph, strep and E. coli infections, diabetes, juvenile rheumatoid arthritis, many childhood cancers, meningitis, pneumonia, urinary tract infections, salmonella, Sudden Infant Death Syndrome (SIDS) as well as lifetime protection from Crohn's Disease, ulcerative colitis, some lymphomas, insulin dependent diabetes, and for girls, breast and ovarian cancer. . . .
>
> Nursing also allows your baby to give germs to you so that your immune system can respond and can synthesize antibodies! This means that if your baby has come in contact with something which you have not, (s)he will pass these germs to you at the next nursing; during that feeding, your body will start to manufacture

antibodies for that particular germ. By the time the next feeding arrives, your entire immune system will be working to provide immunities for you and your baby.[1]

A scientific paper by Melissa Bartick, MD, and Arnold Reinhold:

> [W]e conducted a cost analysis for . . . necrotizing enterocolitis, otitis media, gastroenteritis, hospitalization for lower respiratory tract infections, atopic dermatitis, sudden infant death syndrome, childhood asthma, childhood leukemia, type 1 diabetes mellitus, and childhood obesity. . . .
>
> If 90% of US families could comply with medical recommendations to breastfeed exclusively for 6 months, the United States would save $13 billion per year and prevent an excess 911 deaths, nearly all of which would be in infants ($10.5 billion and 741 deaths at 80% compliance).[2]

When it comes to claims of benefits, though, you can't beat the expansive recitation compiled by Baby-Friendly USA:

> Human milk provides the optimal mix of nutrients and antibodies necessary for each baby to thrive. Scientific studies have shown us that breastfed children have far fewer and less serious illnesses than those who never receive breast milk, including a reduced risk of SIDS, childhood cancers, and diabetes. . . .
>
> Both mother and baby enjoy the emotional benefits of the very special and close relationship formed through breastfeeding. . . .

Families who breastfeed save money. In addition to the fact that breast milk is free, breastfeeding provides savings on health care costs and related time lost to care for sick children. Because breastfeeding saves money, fathers feel less financial pressure and take pride in knowing they are able to give their babies the very best. . . .

When babies are breastfed, both mother and baby are healthier throughout their lives. This translates to lower health care costs and a reduced financial burden on families and third party payers, as well on community and government medical programs.

The environment benefits when babies are breastfed. Scientists agree that breast milk is still the very best way to nourish babies, and may even protect babies from some of the effects of pollution.[3]

If all that were true, calling breast milk the elixir of life would be an understatement.

BREASTFEEDING IS BEST, BUT . . .

One critical fact curiously missing from these amazing claims coming from breastfeeding advocates is that the benefits of breastfeeding differ dramatically between countries with clean water supplies and developing countries where formula is mixed with contaminated water.

Here's the scientific truth about breastfeeding: Breastfeeding has real short-term benefits, but for term infants in countries with reliable clean water supplies, the benefits of breastfeeding are small. That's dramatically different from the claims above. In truth, the notion that breastfeeding is an unparalleled method for ensuring the health of a baby has been promoted by a highly motivated group of activists known as lactivists, who have skillfully and successfully hijacked the public health agenda.

Careful studies show that a population of breastfed infants has an 8 percent decrease in colds and a comparable decrease in diarrheal illnesses in the first year, which for the average infant that means possibly one fewer cold and possibly one fewer episode of diarrheal illness.[4] Extensive reviews of the scientific literature have failed to confirm evidence for a protective effect on obesity, blood pressure, cholesterol levels, diabetes, or IQ.[5] A recent comprehensive study within families shows that most of the purported benefits of breastfeeding disappeared when corrected for race, culture, and socioeconomic factors.[6] So there appears to be no credible, reproducible, scientific evidence that breastfeeding has any long-term health impact.

But just as "natural" birth has become the holy grail of childbirth, breastfeeding has become the holy grail of infant nourishment—at times, ironically, to the detriment of the infant. How did we get to this place? Let's start by taking a deep dive into the scientific evidence about breastfeeding.

THE SCIENTIFIC FACTS VERSUS LACTIVIST CLAIMS

Lactivists cite scientific studies to bolster their claims. Laypeople often assume that because a study is published in a scientific journal, this means that it is true. In reality, the publication of a specific study means it is worthy of being considered in the discussions of that subject. The reason that we have scientific journals in the first place is to allow scientists and physicians to consider the validity of the claims: that is to say, to determine whether the evidence has been analyzed in the proper way, whether the evidence actually shows what the authors claim, and most important, whether the authors have failed to consider alternative explanations for their findings.

At first glance, there seems to be a considerable body of scientific evidence supporting a multitude of short- and long-range benefits to breastfeeding. That's certainly what lactivists believe and aggressively promote. They note that breast milk is known to prevent neonatal enterocolitis (NEC), a severe complication that affects premature infants (it does), and imply that breast milk has similar benefits in term infants (it doesn't).

The list of additional purported benefits is extremely impressive, implying that if you breastfeed your baby you will lower his or her risk of major illness, as well as increase his or her intellectual achievement. Who wouldn't want those advantages for her child? There is a big problem with these claims, though; it is impossible to tell whether the differences in breastfed infants and formula-fed infants are a result of breast milk or simply a reflection of the fact that infants who were breastfed were different in fundamental ways from infants who were not.

Imagine a study comparing two groups of children to determine if breastfeeding increases children's height. Suppose we find that the children from group A, who as infants were exclusively breastfed, turn out to be several inches taller at age five than the children from group B, who never received breast milk.

Should we conclude that breastfeeding made the children in group A taller than the formula-fed children in group B?

It might appear that way at first, but as students of statistics know, you must compare like with like. Are the mothers in group A exactly the same as the mothers in group B?

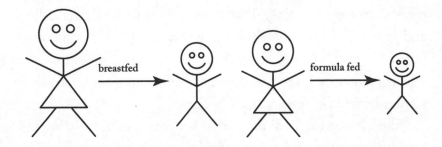

Now we see that the mothers in group A are actually taller than the mothers in group B. We therefore cannot conclude that breastfeeding increased the height of the children. The more likely explanation is that the children in group A are taller than the children in group B because of genetic inheritance. The mothers' height is a confounding variable.

That's the problem that afflicts most of the published literature on the benefits of breastfeeding. We know, for example, that breastfeeding rates in first world countries are closely tied to maternal education, socioeconomic class, and ethnicity.[7] Therefore, observed differences between breastfed babies and formula-fed babies might be due to differences in mothers and environments, not differences in feeding methods. It would not be surprising to find that breastfed babies of women who are college educated and relatively well off and who have access to health insurance and regular pediatric care are healthier than non-breastfed babies who lack these advantages. Breastfeeding has little to do with the difference.

In order for the result of any study comparing breastfeeding to bottle-feeding to be valid, the authors must correct for confounding variables. Most existing studies touting the benefits of breastfeeding have failed to perform this correction.

What happens when you do perform the correction? Most of the purported benefits of breastfeeding as a sole source of nourishment simply disappear, leaving only a small reduction in the risk of colds and diarrheal illness in the first year, as I mentioned earlier.

BREASTFEEDING AND IMMUNITY

Some of the most fanciful claims about the benefits of breast milk concern its role in aiding the newborn immune system. While breastfeeding does provide a boost in preventing infant colds and diarrheal illness, additional claims of immune benefits are quite exaggerated. In order to understand why, we need to understand a bit about the immune system.

The immune system has two major components: cellular immunity and humoral immunity. Cellular immunity is provided by white blood cells that can engulf and destroy harmful bacteria. Humoral immunity encompasses antibodies produced in direct response to contact with bacteria and viruses. There are different types of antibodies of different sizes. The most important type of antibody in breast milk is IgA (immunoglobulin A).[8] IgA can protect mucous membranes (like the lining of the digestive tract and the lining of the respiratory tract) from bacteria and viruses. That's why breastfed babies are less likely to have diarrheal illnesses or colds in the first year.

Most other diseases can be prevented with other types of antibodies. These protective antibodies can cross the placenta from the mother to the baby, but they cannot be passed in breast milk. That's why breastfeeding can't replace vaccination. Even if the mother is immune to whooping cough, for example, she can't pass that immunity to her baby through breast milk. She can pass it through the placenta during pregnancy, but those antibodies will last in the baby's bloodstream for only six months at the longest.

And that's why claims that the mother changes the immunologically active components of breast milk in response to infant disease are highly suspect.

Lactivists make expansive claims, such as those of Katie Hinde, a biologist and associate professor at the Center for Evolution and Medicine at the School of Human Evolution and Social Change at Arizona State University:

> If the mammary gland receptors detect the presence of pathogens, they compel the mother's body to produce antibodies to fight it, and those antibodies travel through breast milk back into the baby's body, where they target the infection.[9]

But supposedly that's not all:

> Even before babies have any concept of time, breast milk helps them understand certain hours from other hours, night from day.
>
> "Milk is so incredibly dynamic," says Hinde. "There are hormones in breast milk, and they reflect the hormones in the mother's circulation. The ones that help facilitate sleep or waking up are present in your milk. And day milk is going to have a completely different hormonal milieu than night milk."

This is yet another example of the exaggerated claims that far, far outstrip the existing scientific evidence.

Hinde and other researchers on breast milk have noted that when babies are sick, the antibody content of breast milk rises. They've proposed an extraordinary mechanism for how babies communicate to their mother that they are sick. Their theory is known as "spit backwash." Baby saliva is supposedly sucked into the breast, where the mother's body senses the bacteria or virus and makes antibodies in response.

But there is another far simpler, far more likely explanation. It's hard for two people to be much closer than a mother and her feeding infant. If a baby has a cold, for example, the mother can simply *breathe in* the virus expelled when the baby sneezes and make antibodies to the virus to protect *herself* from the cold. Those antibodies then end up in the breast milk incidentally as a result of being in the mother's bloodstream. If Hinde and her cohorts had looked, they would likely have found that the father and siblings were making the same antibodies as the mother, not to transmit them to the baby, but to protect themselves.

How about the claim that breast milk helps facilitate infant sleep?

Yes, there are sleep-promoting compounds in breast milk produced at night, but that doesn't mean they are there to help the baby sleep. They may be there simply because the mother is tired. In other words, the presence of these compounds is incidental. Is it possible that they induce sleep in the infant? It's possible but not particularly likely, since babies have their own sleep patterns that are, as any new mother could tell you, sadly unrelated to their mothers' need and desire for sleep.

Do babies communicate their immunological and sleep needs through breast milk? At the moment, there's no evidence to support that view. There are far simpler explanations for the presence of antibodies and other bioactive compounds in breast milk than spit backwash. They are created by the mother to protect the mother. Any benefit to the baby has yet to be demonstrated.

THE MOST COMPREHENSIVE STUDY OF BREASTFEEDING BENEFITS THUS FAR

The 2014 study "Is Breast Truly Best? Estimating the Effects of Breastfeeding on Long-Term Child Health and Wellbeing in the United States Using Sibling Comparisons"[10] by Cynthia Colen and David Ramey confirms what the scientific evidence in large populations has shown all along. The benefits of breastfeeding are trivial.

In many ways, this is the study that we have been waiting for. The study looked at breastfeeding versus bottle-feeding between babies, between families who breastfed or bottle-fed all the children in the family, and most important, *within* families by comparing siblings who were fed differently, thereby eliminating the influence of ethnicity, maternal education, and socioeconomic class.

What did the authors find?

There were differences between breastfed and bottle-fed children in ten of the eleven measured variables when looking at the overall group. Those differences persisted when comparing families in which all the children were breastfed to families where all the children were bottle-fed. But when the authors looked *within* families, there was no significant difference between breastfed and bottle-fed children.

Here is a modified version of the table they presented:

Unadjusted Means and (Sample Sizes) for Select Child Wellbeing Outcomes by Breastfeeding Status (Yes/No),
1986–2010: All NLSY Children and Sibling Subsamples.

	Full Sample[a]		Sibling Sample[b]		Discordant Sibling Sample[b]	
	Breastfed	Not Breastfed	Breastfed	Not Breastfed	Breastfed	Not Breastfed
Body Mass Index	17.83	18.55	17.78	18.47	18.40	18.59
Obesity (%)	11.91	17.38	11.63	17.03	16.36	18.14
Asthma (%)	7.91	6.79	7.43	6.40	7.95	8.89
Hyperactivity Score[c]	101.79	104.68	101.91	104.47	102.97	103.81
Parental Attachment	19.94	19.29	20.04	19.39	19.68	19.54
Behavioral Compliance	25.19	24.65	25.23	24.67	24.93	24.88
PIAT Math Skills[c]	106.87	100.11	107.11	100.38	102.39	101.06
PIAT Reading Recognition[c]	109.36	103.35	109.58	103.43	106.30	104.81
Peabody Picture Vocabulary Test[c]	100.40	90.43	100.91	90.97	94.54	93.26
Weschler Intelligence Scale (WISC)[c]	10.38	9.58 (8,122)	10.38	9.55 (7,287)	9.91 (1,579)	9.61 (1,666)
Scholastic Competence	178.63	169.39	178.49	169.05	173.27	169.84

Notes: All data are weighted to reflect the complex sampling design of the NLSY79 study.

***$p<0.001$; **$p<0.01$; *$p<0.05$; +$p<0.10$.

a   The full sample is weighted using longitudinal custom probability weights provided by the NLSY.

b   We calculate weights for the sibling sample by dividing the average custom weight of all siblings within a given family by the total number of siblings from that family.

c   Dependent variables are standardized by age.

Source: National Longitudinal Survey of Youth, 1979—Children's Sample (NLSY–Childrens).

Simply put, looking within families takes ethnic, cultural, and socioeconomic factors out of the picture. When you do that, you find virtually *no difference* between breastfed and bottle-fed children. In other words, the benefits of breastfeeding have been dramatically overstated, and it is time to correct our advice to mothers to reflect the real benefits of breastfeeding so as to eliminate the guilt that women currently experience if breastfeeding isn't successful.

ARE THERE LONG-TERM BENEFITS TO BREASTFEEDING?

The World Health Organization published "Long-Term Effects of Breastfeeding: A Systematic Review"[11] by Horta and Victora in 2013. It is a 74-page paper, but it can be summed up in one sentence:

There is no evidence for any long-term health benefits of breastfeeding.

The paper is an evaluation of the entire world literature on the long-term benefits of breastfeeding and it is divided into individual sections for each purported benefit. These include overweight and obesity, blood pressure, serum cholesterol, type 2 diabetes, and intellectual performance.

These results are not surprising. With the exception of IQ testing, the studied outcomes are risk factors for diseases of adulthood and old age. Throughout most of human existence, human life-span was approximately thirty-five years, and diseases of old age had little to no impact on the survival of the species. There is no reason to expect there would be much of an evolutionary advantage to avoiding the diseases of old age. The winners in the sweepstakes of evolution are those who can produce offspring who survive to adulthood and produce more offspring. Obesity was rare and people often didn't live long enough to develop heart disease or diabetes. Therefore, there was no evolutionary benefit to breast milk that would prevent those problems.

In industrialized societies, the benefits of breastfeeding are small and short-term. That's why there is no reason for any mother who chooses bottle-feeding to feel guilty. Breast milk is not "liquid gold." It's just milk and confers a few small, short-term benefits compared to infant formula.

ONE BOTTLE OF FORMULA HARMS BABIES?

Breastfeeding and bottle-feeding are often presented as mutually exclusive, but many women breastfeed and bottle-feed, a practice known as combination (combo) feeding. They do so for many reasons: some women have an insufficient milk supply; some women leave formula for their babies when they go to work so they won't have to take the time to pump; and some women simply want the option of having Dad or another family member feed the baby. Small amounts of formula can even help in establishing a breastfeeding relationship when a baby is losing weight or becoming dehydrated before the mother's milk is in.[12] Unfortunately, as lactivists have become more ideologically rigid, they have begun to rail against any supplementation with formula, regardless of the reason.

Just as lactivists have dramatically exaggerated the benefits of breastfeeding, they have similarly exaggerated the harms of formula-feeding. Their latest efforts center on the infant microbiome, and the biggest canard currently making the rounds is that even one bottle of formula harms babies.

We have already discussed the ways that the natural childbirth advocates have appropriated and misrepresented the emerging information about the infant gut microbiome to demonize C-sections. They got the idea from the lactivists who have taken the same preliminary information and used it to demonize infant formula.

A case in point is "What's Really Wrong with One Bottle:

Microbiota & Metabolic Syndrome."[13] Spoiler alert: What's really wrong with one bottle of infant formula? Absolutely nothing! That's what the scientific evidence tells us.

So if there's nothing wrong with one bottle of infant formula, what does Dr. Lawrence Noble talk about? I've reviewed all eighty-three slides in one of his talks and not one of them shows any evidence that a single bottle of formula causes any impact at all, let alone a harmful impact. Imagine if we tried to address smoking-related illness by humiliating anyone who ever had one cigarette. Imagine if we tried to address obesity by shaming anyone who ever ate even once at McDonald's. That's absurd, right? But that's the equivalent of what the lactivists are doing.

PROMOTING MOTHER-INFANT BONDING

One of the primary reasons that women give for deciding to breastfeed is the belief that it promotes mother-infant bonding. Breastfeeding advocates have emphasized this point for years. Curiously, there is no evidence in the scientific literature on children and attachment that feeding method has any impact at all on bonding. As we shall see, mother-infant bonding appears to be mediated by the child's belief that the mother can meet his or her needs for food, care, and emotional support, not by the specific methods by which these needs are met. Do mothers who hold their adopted newborns for the first time feel any less bonded to them because they cannot breastfeed them? I think any adoptive mother would certainly dismiss that statement out of hand.

In "Breastfeeding and Maternal Mental and Physical Health,"[14] a chapter in the book *Women's Health Psychology*, Jennifer Hahn-Holbrook and her colleagues supply an exhaustive review of the existing literature. The authors appear to strongly favor breastfeeding, but even they have to admit:

> Conventional wisdom holds that breastfeeding helps mothers bond with their babies. In fact, one of the most common reasons given by women for wanting to breastfeed is the opportunity to bond with their children. In the scientific literature as well, breastfeeding is often assumed to aid in maternal-infant attachment, without necessarily giving reference to direct evidence. Given this, it is surprising that only a few studies have actually tested this hypothesis in humans, and even fewer have found significant results.

So if there's no evidence that breastfeeding promotes bonding, where did the idea come from? Breastfeeding advocates simply made it up.

In the absence of any evidence to support the claim, why has it been promoted so vigorously and so widely? It is just another variation of the efforts to moralize childbirth and child care.

OTHERS HAVE POINTED OUT EXAGGERATION OF BENEFITS

The scientific evidence for the bulk of the purported benefits of breastfeeding has always been weak, conflicting, and riddled with confounders. This has been known for decades, but those who have pointed it out have been shouted down.

Joan Wolf of Texas A&M University provided a spot-on description of the tendency of lactivists to exaggerate breastfeeding's benefits far out of proportion to the scientific evidence. In a

2007 paper entitled "Is Breast Really Best? Risk and Total Motherhood in the National Breastfeeding Awareness Campaign"[15]
(subsequently expanded into a book[16] published in 2011), she
describes the fear-mongering tactics of lactivists:

> From June 2004 to April 2006, cosponsored by the U.S.
> Department of Health and Human Services and the Ad
> Council, the National Breastfeeding Awareness Cam-
> paign (NBAC) warned women that not breast-feeding
> put babies at risk for a variety of health problems.
> "You'd never take risks before your baby is born. Why
> start after?" asked televised public service announce-
> ments over images of pregnant women logrolling and
> riding a mechanical bull. . . . The campaign was based
> on research that is inconsistent, lacks strong associa-
> tions, and does not account for plausible confounding
> variables, such as the role of parental behavior, in vari-
> ous health outcomes. It capitalized on public misun-
> derstanding of risk and risk assessment by portraying
> infant nutrition as a matter of safety versus danger and
> then creating spurious analogies.

In light of the known scientific evidence, that the benefits of
breastfeeding in first world countries are small, Wolf questions
the ethical obligations of those who wish to promote breastfeeding. Is their moralizing justified by the scientific evidence? Is the
scientific evidence being presented accurately? Do public health
officials have ethical obligations to be truthful?

> Medical journals are replete with contradictory conclu-
> sions about the impact of breast-feeding: for every study
> linking it to better health, another finds it to be irrel-

evant, weakly significant, or inextricably tied to other unmeasured or unmeasurable factors. While many of these investigations describe a correlation between breast-feeding and more desirable outcomes, the notion that breast-feeding itself contributes to better health is far less certain, and this is a crucial distinction that breast-feeding proponents have consistently elided.

Wolf's work was a scholarly treatment. Hanna Rosin evoked a far greater outcry with her 2009 *Atlantic* magazine piece "The Case Against Breast-feeding."[17] She too tackles the scientific literature and concludes:

> We have clear indications that breast-feeding helps prevent an extra incident of gastrointestinal illness in some kids—an unpleasant few days of diarrhea or vomiting, but rarely life-threatening in developed countries. We have murky correlations with a whole bunch of long-term conditions. The evidence on IQs is intriguing but not all that compelling. . . .
>
> So overall, yes, breast is probably best. But not so much better that formula deserves the label of "public health menace," alongside smoking. Given what we know so far, it seems reasonable to put breast-feeding's health benefits on the plus side of the ledger and other things—modesty, independence, career, sanity—on the minus side, and then tally them up and make a decision. But in this risk-averse age of parenting, that's not how it's done.

Rosin successfully and (mostly) happily breastfed her own children. You might think that would have protected her from backlash, but you would be wrong. Writing in the *Chicago Tribune*, Judith Graham insists:

> The author is sloppy. . . .
>
> "Unfortunately, she drew conclusions from a hasty scan of a few selected references and didn't mention a large body of powerful evidence supporting breast-feeding," said Dr. Ruth Lawrence, chair of the pediatric academy's section on breast-feeding. . . .
>
> Rosin's real gripe is that the benefits of breast-feeding have been oversold, making moms guilty if they chose to feed their babies formula. . . .
>
> [T]he guilt and the angst over whether or not to breast-feed is her problem, as is her perception that she'll be less than an uber-mom if she gives her baby a bottle. Who told her she had to be an uber-mom, anyway?[18]

Jennifer Block, writing for *Babble*,[19] acknowledges that lactivist campaigns may have overstated the benefits of breastfeeding—and then proceeds to overstate the benefits of breastfeeding:

> [B]reastfeeding PSAs have shamelessly sunk to playing the bad mother card (see ad that likens formula-feeding to riding a mechanical bull while pregnant). No, formula is not poison. It is a lifesaving intervention when needed, much like the C-section. A satisfactory substitute. The problem is that it should never have come to be seen as equivalent to normal physiology, the superiority of which is really quite breathtaking when you think about it.

But the central point of Rosin's piece is that the purported superiority of breastfeeding *isn't* breathtaking at all; it's negligible.

BREASTFEEDING IS HARD

In recent years, more than 75 percent of new mothers started breastfeeding before leaving the hospital, yet less than 38 percent were exclusively breastfeeding at three months, and only 16.4 percent were exclusively breastfeeding at six months.[20] Why is there such a tremendous gulf between maternal aspirations and practice? Because breastfeeding can be incredibly difficult, a lot harder than breastfeeding advocates acknowledge.

Breastfeeding advocates propose that women stop breastfeeding because hospitals give out formula or because of lack of education, professional support, peer support, or dedication to the process. All this pretending reflects the profound unwillingness of breastfeeding advocates to acknowledge the real reasons that women stop breastfeeding or fail to start in the first place. The dirty little secret about breastfeeding is that starting is difficult, often painful, frustrating, and sometimes onerous. And continuing breastfeeding is hard, sometimes painful, and not always practical, especially for women who work, which in 2016 are most women. Moreover, breastfeeding, like pregnancy, is not perfect. Just as 20 percent of established pregnancies will end in miscarriage, a significant percentage of breastfeeding mothers will not be able to produce enough to completely nourish their babies with breast milk alone.[21]

What are the reasons for being unable to produce enough breast milk to completely support a baby? There are two types of causes, primary and secondary. Primary causes include "insufficient mammary glandular tissue, postpartum hemorrhage with

Sheehan syndrome, theca lutein cyst, polycystic ovarian syndrome, and some breast surgeries."

Secondary causes include a baby's inability to feed (decreased muscle tone, cleft palate) or poor breastfeeding technique.

Breastfeeding advocates insist on eliding or burying these difficulties. And because they insist on ignoring the experiences of women, their well-meaning attempts at encouraging extended breastfeeding are almost complete failures. I'm not sure why breastfeeding activists refuse to acknowledge the reality of breastfeeding. They prefer to present ideas like "breast milk is always available," "breast milk is always the perfect temperature," and "breast feeding saves money." Those statements may be true, but they ignore the very real challenges in initiating and maintaining breastfeeding.

Perhaps breastfeeding activists fear that women will not attempt breastfeeding if they are informed honestly about the difficulties. Yet it appears that the opposite is true. By not acknowledging these difficulties ahead of time, breastfeeding activists set women up for failure. Breastfeeding is a learned behavior. It is not instinctual on the part of the mother, and although a baby has the instinct to suckle, latching on properly and actually getting milk requires practice. A new mother and a new baby may get frustrated very quickly when things do not proceed smoothly. Let's take a look at Moira.

Moira's daughter would not stop crying:

Two days later, my daughter had lost over 10 percent of her body weight. She screamed inconsolably between multiple-hour-long nursing sessions which never left her satisfied; she'd fall into an exhausted sleep for perhaps twenty minutes, then wake up to scream and nurse for hours again. The nurses told me this was normal; the lactation consultants told me over and over again

that I just needed to keep offering her the breast (I hadn't show-
ered in over seventy-two hours because she was on the breast
all the time, but somehow she wasn't being offered the breast
enough?) and that I should pump when she wasn't nursing to
build up my supply. By the third day, our very pro-breastfeeding
pediatrician told me to supplement so that she could gain enough
weight back to go home. . . . Insanely, the LC I saw later that
day, after my daughter had fallen into her first contented deep
sleep following (shockingly enough) her first real feed, was visibly
disappointed that I'd "given up" by feeding my daughter formula
after she'd nursed and screamed for hours that afternoon.

New mothers are often emotionally fragile, due to the effect of
hormones. A baby screaming desperately in hunger (and all babies
begin to scream desperately within seconds of realizing they are
hungry) can upset even an experienced mother. It's much worse
for a new and inexperienced mother who desperately wants to satisfy the baby, fearing that the baby is starving. Prior to the advent
of formula, if you were wealthy you could hire a wet nurse, but for
everyone else there was no choice but to stick with the first inexperienced attempts and keep going. Now, with formula at hand
and able to satisfy an infant in seconds, it may seem pointless or
even cruel (not to mention harrowing to the mother) to force a
baby to figure out breastfeeding if it isn't coming easily.

Initiating breastfeeding is often painful. Cracked and bleeding nipples are every bit as unpleasant as they sound. Countless
new mothers tell stories of bursting into tears whenever the baby
starts to cry, in anticipation of the pain of nursing.

Gem remembers:

My son was alert and very interested in breastfeeding. The nurse
and our doula both agreed it looked like he was latched correctly.

It was very uncomfortable for me, but having never actually breastfed before, I wasn't sure what was normal. By the second day in the hospital, my nipples were bleeding. Everyone, including the hospital lactation consultant, kept assuring me my son was latched correctly.

For most women, the pain disappears over time, but it can take days or even weeks. Breastfeeding advocates blame mothers themselves for this pain, insisting that they are positioning the baby in the wrong way. The truth is that women can do everything right and still have this pain. It simply has to be ignored until it goes away, and it is hardly surprising that some women do not want to wait that long.

Maintaining breastfeeding while working is also incredibly difficult. During the typical workday, a woman may need to pump twice or more times, each session taking twenty to thirty minutes and requiring a clean and private space, a breast pump, and a refrigerator to store the milk. Professional women may be able to assemble these resources, but the average working woman in the average work environment may not have the access to such things or the time to pump on the job. That is just reality.

The demographics of breastfeeding reflect the difficulties. Breastfeeding is associated with higher levels of maternal education and higher income levels.[22] Women of color and women of lower socioeconomic status are far less likely to breastfeed than their well-off white peers. Economic success makes it easier to continue breastfeeding because women may not have to work, may enjoy extended maternity leaves, may have private space at the workplace in which to pump, and can afford high-quality equipment.

Should we encourage breastfeeding? Of course, but not to the detriment of maternal and baby well-being.

INSUFFICIENT BREAST MILK

Here is Lisa's story:

> *I discovered, after having my first child, that I didn't have enough ductile tissue to make an adequate amount of milk for my son. Because everything I read proclaimed the supremacy of breast milk, I took fenugreek capsules, drank water almost obsessively, and pumped every time I nursed. I also convinced myself, possibly influenced by all the sleep I wasn't getting while pumping and washing pump parts and extra bottles, that I was not meant to be a mother and that my baby would be better off with someone else. I spent a lot of my baby's first year pondering how to kill myself and make it look like an accident, and wondering whether my husband would be able to attract a new wife soon enough to give my son a sibling.*

Mothers are not the only ones who suffer from the relentless effort to promote breastfeeding. Babies suffer too. The promotion of breastfeeding invariably involves discussion of the benefits to babies of breast milk, but there seems to be little concern for the babies who suffer in an attempt to force them to breastfeed even when the breastfeeding relationship is not working—for example, if the mother is not able to produce enough breast milk.

Hunger is probably the most elemental of infant drives and, as anyone who has seen an infant scream from hunger would probably agree, is experienced by the baby as suffering. For most mothers, myself included, the sound of their own infant crying is piercing in its intensity and distress. I remember being surprised by this when my first child was born. I had spent my entire professional life surrounded by crying babies and it had never bothered me, yet I found my son's crying unbearable and always rushed to determine what was wrong and fix it in any way possible. I cannot imagine letting any of my infants cry in hunger for any length of time without feeding them. Indeed, I recoil when I read about the infant care manuals of the early twentieth century, which advised mothers to feed the baby on a schedule designed for maternal convenience instead of infant needs.

So why do lactivists advise women that insufficient milk supply is a "myth"? According to Jack Newman, MD, considered an international expert on breastfeeding:

> The vast majority of women produce more than enough milk. Indeed, an overabundance of milk is common. Most babies that gain too slowly, or lose weight, do so not because the mother does not have enough milk, but because the baby does not get the milk that the mother has. The usual reason that the baby does not get the milk that is available is that he is poorly latched onto the breast.[23]

The first step is to blame yourself or your baby or both. And what if your baby truly is not getting enough milk? Dr. Newman recommends no less than seven different strategies, tried over several *days*, before supplementing with infant formula:

> Sometimes applying this Protocol for a few days and continuing with it will get the baby gaining more rapidly. Sometimes more rapid growth is necessary and it may not be possible without supplementation. If practical, get banked breast milk to use as a supplement. If not available, infant formula may be necessary.[24]

The second step is to spend days trying to increase your milk supply. Let your baby suffer in the meantime.

Dr. Newman believes that when your pediatrician tells you he or she is concerned that the baby is not gaining enough weight, you should doubt your pediatrician. He argues that "many physicians are too much enamoured with scales. A scale that is properly calibrated (many are not) is true only to itself, not to other scales."[25]

So the third step is to ignore your pediatrician.

Physicians have a name for the series of steps that Dr. Newman recommends: benign neglect. I guess the theory is that if the baby is truly starving, it will eventually become indisputable. Of course the baby could suffer seizures and die of dehydration during that time, but that happens only in the most extreme cases. Dr. Newman apparently believes that as long as the baby does not die, his or her suffering during that time is less important than avoiding infant formula.

That's both heartless and ignores the actual scientific evidence.

It seems to me that one of the biggest ironies of all is when lactivists promote exclusive breastfeeding as "baby-friendly." How could anything that ignores infant suffering be considered baby friendly? It is nonsensical.

THE LACTIVIST RESPONSE TO EVERY BREASTFEEDING PROBLEM: BREASTFEED HARDER

Over the years, I've heard a lot about the physical and mental gymnastics some new mothers put themselves through in order to breastfeed. I often hear about women who breastfeed every two hours, plus use a supplemental nursing system (SNS), plus pump their breasts afterward to further stimulate milk production, typically on the advice of a lactation consultant who may never have personally experienced the problem of insufficient milk supply.

Have lactation consultants lost their minds? Their "advice" is barbaric, and is not in any way justified by scientific evidence. It is especially cruel to women who have a primary cause for failure to produce enough milk. No amount of pumping will change the situation if a woman does not have enough glandular tissue to create breast milk, or has a hormonal problem prohibiting or limiting the production of breast milk.

Adrienne reminds us that mothers aren't the only ones who suffer:

> *I kept up a rigorous schedule of feeding and pumping for months. I felt like it would have been selfish for me to back off, that it didn't matter how tired I was (emotionally, mentally, and physically), that being a good mom meant I had to give him every drop of breast milk that I could. Finally, one day when my son was six or seven months old, my daughter broke down crying. She asked me why I never spent any time with her anymore and why I didn't love her anymore. My desperation to exclusively breastfeed had not only hurt my son, but it had hurt my daughter as well; not only had I been blind to my son's suffering, I had also been blind to my daughter's.*
>
> *The message you always get from lactivists is that breastfeeding makes you a good mom and not breastfeeding makes you an inferior mom, that breast is always best. If "breast is always best," how could striving to exclusively breastfeed hurt either of my children? So, if it was hurting my children, maybe breast isn't always best after all. Maybe what is best is dependent on the situation.*

Sure, all things being equal, breastfeeding is best, but then all things being equal, naturally occurring 20/20 vision is best too. In real life, what's best isn't necessarily what happens. Eyes may be perfectly designed to see 20/20, but fully 30 percent of Americans are nearsighted.[26] That's why we have glasses and contacts. They are not ideal when compared with naturally occurring 20/20 vision, but they are close enough that it really doesn't matter.

Similarly, in real life, breasts may be perfectly designed to provide adequate breast milk, but 5 percent or more of women don't make adequate milk. That's why we have formula. Though formula is not ideal when compared to natural occurring exclusive breastfeeding, it is close enough that *it really doesn't matter!*

Moreover, new motherhood is hard! It is a tremendous physical and emotional adjustment, compounded by hormonal changes that can lead to the "baby blues" or true postpartum depression.

If we want to support new mothers, and we claim that we do, we should be supporting their physical recovery and emotional adjustment. That means ensuring that they get enough sleep to fully heal, enough support with all aspects of mothering to feel competent, and enough reassurance that the most important thing each baby needs is maternal love, not breast milk.

The sad fact is that these people and programs that support exclusive breastfeeding are not supporting new mothers, they are supporting the breastfeeding industry, with its consultants, equipment, supplements, and aids. And in their near-religious devotion to the idea of breastfeeding, they are cruel to mothers and babies.

THE BABY-FRIENDLY HOSPITAL INITIATIVE

The Baby-Friendly Hospital Initiative (BFHI) was launched by the World Health Organization and United Nations Children's

Fund (UNICEF) in 1991 to encourage breastfeeding. The BFHI credential is given to hospitals that follow ten specific steps in caring for women after they've given birth.[27] These include:

- Inform all pregnant women about the benefits and management of breastfeeding.
- Help mothers initiate breastfeeding within one hour of birth.
- Give infants no food or drink other than breast milk, unless medically indicated.
- Practice rooming in—allow mothers and infants to remain together twenty-four hours a day.
- Give no pacifiers or artificial nipples to breastfeeding infants.

All newborns must room in in order to support breastfeeding? How can a new mother get desperately needed sleep if she isn't allowed to hand her baby off to professionals for a few hours? She can't.

Give no food or drink other than breast milk? Some hospitals actually take this further and lock up the formula.[28] How can a mother soothe a baby screaming from hunger before he or she learns to nurse effectively if she doesn't have access to formula? In many cases she can't, and she becomes frantic with anxiety even before she leaves the hospital. That's cruel.

Every woman must be informed of the benefits of breastfeeding? Why? Did her right to control her own body come out with the placenta? It's no one's business whether a woman breastfeeds except her own. Anything else is profoundly anti-feminist.

And when she leaves the BFHI hospital?

Every woman must exclusively feed breast milk, and must engage in an endless cycle of feeding, combined with SNS and pumping? It places the value of breast milk above a woman's emotional and physical health and her ability to bond with her baby. And it essentially traps a woman in the home, nursing, for the entirety of the day. For some women, this prescription is unbearable!

There are so many people to blame for this extremism that it's difficult to know where to begin. Obviously lactation consultants and lactivist organizations like the Baby Friendly Hospital Initiative bear the brunt of the blame. It's business for them, and they put the health of their business ahead of the health of their patients, both babies and mothers.

But there's plenty of blame to go around. Many physicians have elevated breastfeeding too, going far, far beyond what the scientific evidence shows. Many research scientists start their research papers with the conclusion that breastfeeding must be encouraged and that women should receive more breastfeeding support (in other words, more business for the lactivist industry) and simply ignore the actual findings that show that while breastfeeding has beneficial effects, in industrialized countries, those benefits are trivial. This happens because of phenomenon known as white hat bias.[29]

According to the researchers who first described it:

> "White hat bias" . . . lead[s] to distortion of information in the service of what may be perceived to be righteous ends. . . . WHB may be conjectured to be fuelled by feelings of righteous zeal, indignation toward certain aspects of industry, or other factors.

One of the first described cases of white hat bias was the promotion of breastfeeding. The indignation is the result of the reprehensible conduct of formula manufacturers in the developing world. In an effort to increase market share, companies like Nestlé promoted formula in countries that lacked clean water supplies. The result was a tragedy that was easily foreseeable. Babies died because their mothers replaced breast milk with formula mixed with contaminated water.

As Suzanne Barston explains in *Bottled Up*,[30] the actions of formula manufacturers

> have caused a reverse halo effect, making it difficult for some to separate the product from the producer. Formula as a substance did not convince women that their bodies weren't capable of nurturing life; marketing executives, injustices, and bad circumstances did a bang-up job of that all on their own. Formula as a substance does not kill babies; the water used to reconstitute it does—rather than blame the powder sitting in the can, we should be blaming the infrastructure.

In other words, formula has been demonized partly because of disgust with formula manufacturers. White hat bias leads researchers to tout the superiority of breast milk far beyond what the actual research shows. As a result, public health officials have gotten far out in front of the scientific evidence, grossly exaggerating the benefits and importance of breastfeeding and using weak, contradictory data riddled with confounding variables to do so.

Let's finish with what I consider the most important baseline reality. The key to a healthy, happy, thriving infant is a physically and emotionally healthy mother. That means a mother who is getting enough rest, whose mental health needs are being addressed, and who is able to enjoy substantial amounts of time happily bonding with her child.

Breast milk is not essential and is not necessarily best for every mother-infant pair, and the effort to produce it is absolutely harmful in some situations. All of the madness around breastfeeding begs the question: Do we care about mothers and babies or do we just care about breast milk?

We've spent millions promoting breastfeeding. Where's the return on investment?

Public health initiatives by definition are meant to improve public health. They are usually based on solid scientific evidence; their implementation saves thousands, if not millions, of lives; and they pay for themselves many times over in lives saved, earnings preserved, and medical expenditures averted. We have spent millions of dollars promoting vaccination and supporting efforts to stop smoking, and these actions have paid off in both lives and money saved.

Breastfeeding initiation rates have tripled since 1970 rising from 25 percent to 75 percent. So where is the return on investment?

In the United States, the rate of breastfeeding initiation has varied dramatically over the last hundred years.[31] Because of this variation, we have an excellent opportunity to determine whether those purported benefits really occur across populations and over time.

How has breastfeeding affected various measures of health in our country? Let's look first at infant mortality rates in comparison to the popularity of breastfeeding.

According to the CDC, there was a precipitous decline in infant mortality over the course of the twentieth century. During that time the breastfeeding initiation rate dropped from nearly 100% in 1900 to a low of 24% in 1970, only to rebound to 71% by 2000; the infant mortality rate declined steadily throughout.

Life expectancy has risen over steadily over the twentieth century and breastfeeding rates appear to have had no effect on the rise.

What about IQ?

American IQ has risen 25 points in a linear fashion from 1915 to 2000,[32] and once again breastfeeding rates appear to have had no impact.

In other words, there is no effect of breastfeeding initiation rates on infant mortality, life expectancy, or IQ.

Obviously, there were other factors at work in improving health and IQ than breastfeeding, including better medical care, better nutrition, and better education. And the decline in infant mortality is due to the improvement in obstetrics and the use of medical interventions, as discussed in previous chapters.

But where is the evidence that thousands of lives have been saved by breastfeeding? Where is the evidence that millions of cases of disease have been prevented? Where is the evidence of millions of dollars in health-care expenditures averted? Where is the evidence that the dramatic rise in breastfeeding has had any impact at all on infant or child health?

This doesn't mean that breastfeeding is a bad thing. To the contrary, it's a good thing, but the benefits for children in first world countries are trivial. If those benefits were anything other than trivial, we should have seen a dramatic impact on infant health and pediatric care expenditure in the past forty-five years when breastfeeding initiation rates rose by 200 percent, but we haven't seen anything of the kind.

Unless, of course, you count the soul-searing guilt and feelings of inadequacy among women who can't or choose not to breastfeed.

A BLUEPRINT FOR SHAMING FORMULA FEEDERS

Erin's pain is palpable:

> *I tried to breastfeed. I tried really hard. I don't know why I need to underline that, but I do. He had IUGR [intrauterine growth restriction] and a high palate. I'm not sure he ever latched on for more than comfort. I couldn't make enough milk, and I had to give him formula. I had a C-section and they wouldn't let me see him until the next day. That was the first of my failures in mothering. I couldn't breastfeed. I pumped until he was eleven months old. The day I stopped, I tried to kill myself.*
>
> *There's a reasonable part of me that knows that what matters is my baby is healthy and well fed. He is. I'm certain of it. But another part says that I'm garbage. I'm a failure. I'm lazy and ignorant and a lousy mother.*

Sadly, shame seems to be integral to the contemporary lactivism movement. Indeed, it is so integral that there's an actual blueprint on how lactivists can shame other mothers. Entitled "Watch Your Language," it was written by lactation consultant Diane Wiessinger and published in the *Journal of Human Lactation* in 1996.[33] It is a primer on how to mobilize language to shame women who bottle-feed.

Wiessinger identifies the problem for those wishing to shame mothers. Merely telling them that "breast is best" leaves open the possibility that you can still be a good mother if you formula-feed (though in Wiessinger's parlance, this is referred to as artificial feeding):

> When we . . . say that breastfeeding is the best possible way to feed babies because it provides their ideal food,

perfectly balanced for optimal infant nutrition, the logical response is, "So what?" Our own experience tells
us that optimal is not necessary. Normal is fine, and
implied in this language is the absolute normalcy—and
thus safety and adequacy—of artificial feeding. . . .

Artificial feeding, which is neither the same nor
superior, is therefore deficient, incomplete, and inferior.
Those are difficult words, but they have an appropriate
place in our vocabulary.

Actually, they are ugly, shaming words, and Wiessinger is just
getting started:

Because breastfeeding is the biological norm, breastfed babies are not "healthier"; artificially fed babies are
ill more often and more seriously. Breastfed babies do
not "smell better"; artificial feeding results in an abnormal and unpleasant odor that reflects problems in the
infant's gut.

Wiessinger insists:

When we fail to describe the hazards of artificial feeding, we deprive mothers of crucial decision-making
information. The mother having difficulty with breastfeeding may not seek help just to achieve a "special
bonus"; but she may clamor for help if she knows how
much she and her baby stand to lose. She is less likely
to use artificial baby milk just "to get him used to a
bottle" if she knows that the contents of that bottle
cause harm.

Why would anyone undertake shame as a deliberate effort to promote breastfeeding? For Wiessinger, it isn't about babies or mothers; it's about promoting a "breastfeeding culture."

> We cannot expect to create a breastfeeding culture if we do not insist on a breastfeeding model of health in both our language and our literature.

Over the past twenty years Wiessinger's dream of using shaming language to browbeat women into breastfeeding has come true. The breastfeeding initiation rate has reached a hundred-year high. And as noted earlier, the impact on infant health has been negligible to nonexistent. In contrast, the impact on maternal mental health has been profound. Simply put, this has resulted in an epidemic of guilty mothers who are ashamed that they cannot breastfeed exclusively.

The authors of a recent paper, "Shame If You Do—Shame If You Don't," explain:

> In many cultures, breastfeeding is synonymous with 'good mothering.' . . . When mothers make a decision not to breastfeed, they may experience guilt, blame and feelings of failure. . . . [F]ormula feeding mothers may experience shame (as opposed to guilt) through 'failure' to live up to ideals of womanhood and motherhood.[34]

So if babies don't benefit in any measurable way from breastfeeding promotion through shaming and mothers are actually harmed by it, who does benefit?

First, lactation consultants benefit by increased employment opportunities and income. If every women is shamed into attempting breastfeeding, and shamed if she attempts to stop, and shamed if she combo-feeds with formula, and shamed when she is seen bottle-feeding, there will be a greater need for lactation consultants.

Second, lactivists benefit in the same way that those inflicting shame on others always benefit, by enhanced self-esteem through feeling superior to the shamed.

Finally, lactivists benefit by enjoying ugly behavior that is usually forbidden but is actually encouraged in the case of formula-feeding. There is simply no limit to the cruelty of lactivists toward women who don't or don't want to breastfeed, and no limit to the delight that lactivists experience in sanctioned cruelty toward other mothers.

LACTIVISM AND CRUELTY

In *The Washington Post* in October 2014, Emily Wax-Thibodeaux felt compelled to explain why she didn't breastfeed.[35] Wax-Thibodeaux recounted her experience with lactation consultants who harassed and shamed her after the birth of her son despite the fact that she had undergone a double mastectomy for breast cancer!

Five years after the operation that saved her life:

> We were cleared to try getting pregnant. But because chemotherapy ravages fertility and I was now 37, we found ourselves saving money and signing up for in vitro fertilization.
>
> Jan. 29, 2014, I gave birth to a 7½-pound baby boy.
>
> "You never gave up," my husband said, laughing as he

watched Lincoln gulp down his first two-ounce serving of formula, which my husband fed to him.

As the two of them cuddled afterward, I was in a mood that I can describe only as postpartum elation.

That is, until those I jokingly call the "breast-feeding Nazis" came marching in to my room.

Despite her medical history:

"You really should breast-feed," the hospital's lactation consultants, a.k.a. "lactivists," said.

When I simply said, "I'm going to do formula," they didn't want to leave it at that.

So holding my day-old newborn on what was one of the most blissful days of my life, I had to tell the aggressive band of well-intentioned strangers my whole cancer saga.

"Just try," they advised. "Let's hope you get some milk."

"It may come out anyway, or through your armpits," another advised later.

These are supposed health professionals. Their ignorance is astounding—mastectomy removes all breast tissue, even the tail of the breast that extends into the armpit.

Unfortunately, shaming is integral to lactivism because shaming others is integral to the self-image of lactivists. All their so-called baby-friendly initiatives aren't actually friendly to babies, and they certainly aren't friendly to mothers; they are friendly only to lactivists.

The shaming and blaming so beloved of lactivists, their

comments, and even many of their "scientific" claims are self-referential. They reflect the need for lactivists and lactation consultants to boost their own self-esteem and business.

But lactivists are not superior to other mothers; they are just women who chose one excellent form of infant nutrition over another excellent form of nutrition. How you feed your baby is irrelevant. Loving your baby is what counts!

< 6 >

There's No Science That Supports Attachment Parenting

I was an attachment parent.

The term didn't exist when my children were small, but I met the criteria: I had vaginal births, I breastfed, and I carried my babies everywhere; I used to joke that I was magnetically attracted to them. We had an open bed policy for babies and for children who were sick or frightened. For most of the time my children were small I worked exclusively at night while they were sleeping or I didn't work at all. My husband and I were not away from the children for more than a weekend for nearly seventeen years.

My husband was an integral partner. There were years when we met at the train station several nights a week, he returning from a day at the office, me heading to the hospital, and we exchanged children from one set of car seats to another set of car seats. We did it because that's what seemed best for us and our children.

At the time I had friends who were parenting the way that we were and friends who were doing things very differently. As my children grew, I met a wide assortment of *their* friends, some who were being raised in ways similar to them and some who were being raised in totally distinct ways. I've had the opportunity to see how my friends' children have turned out and how my children's friends have turned out and I've noticed something important: you can't tell which children were parented in which style.

I've learned that it is not the style of parenting that matters but whether children are loved and whether they know it. It sounds obvious, so how did anyone come to believe otherwise?

THE DOMINANT MOTHERING IDEOLOGY

We like to say that it takes a village to raise a child, but as with so many things, it is far more revealing to watch what we do than to listen to what we say. What we do suggests that we believe that it takes a mother, and only a mother, to successfully raise a child.

The dominant mothering ideology in the United States today is attachment parenting, also known, revealingly, as intensive mothering. It's the dominant ideology not because it is the way that most people parent, but because it is the ideal held by middle- and upper-middle-class mothers who are often highly vocal on the Internet and social media, and the ideal against which women measure their own mothering and that of other women.

This ideology was first described in 1996 by sociologist Sharon Hays in her book *The Cultural Contradictions of Motherhood*:

> Intensive mothering [is] an ideology that holds the individual mother primarily responsible for child-rearing and dictates that the process is to be child-centered, expert-guided, emotionally absorbing, labor-intensive, and financially expensive.[1]

Attachment parenting rests on a number of unstated and unproven assumptions. At the heart of attachment parenting is the fear that a child's attachment to his or her mother is fragile, difficult to form, and easy to break, and requires intensive effort on the part of the mother to maintain. Moreover, attachment parenting advocates insist that the ability of the child to succeed in the world is directly dependent on the quality of a child's attachment to the mother.

This is very different from what came before. For most of recorded history, parenting was nothing more than raising children to adulthood. Now, as Charlotte Faircloth explains:

> By looking at the language of 'parenting', a picture emerges of a growing momentum from the 1970s onwards towards the targeting of parental behaviour as deficient and also 'parenting' as something of a joyless task or 'job', to be conducted under the watchful gaze of experts. . . . [S]tudies of 'parenting' also thus indicate this term is inherently bound up with the idea that people other than parents have special insights that can and should be brought to bear.[2]

Attachment parenting sounds like it has the support of scientific evidence behind it, but nothing could be further from the truth.

Fact: No scientific evidence exists that children's attachment to their mothers is fragile and contingent.

Fact: The scientific evidence indicates the direct opposite! Infants and children will naturally, spontaneously, and fiercely form deep emotional attachments to those who care for them. Children will tolerate extraordinary amounts of abuse and neglect from a caregiver without any harm at all to the attachment. The attachment endures even in the face of considerable threat to the physical and mental health of the child.

So where did attachment parenting come from? It is in large part a religious ideology, popularized by Dr. William Sears and his wife, Martha Sears, RN. The Searses believe that attachment parenting is God's plan for child-rearing. As they explain in their 1997 book, *The Complete Book of Christian Parenting and Child Care*:

> The type of parenting we believe is God's design for the father-mother-child relationship is a style we call "attachment parenting." Our intent in recommending this style of parenting to you is so strong that we have spent more hours in prayerful thought on this topic than on any other topic in this book. . . . We have a deep personal conviction that this is the way God wants His children parented.[3]

What else does God purportedly expect from parents? From husbands:

> God has given the husband the prime responsibility for making the marriage relationship work, which is as it should be since he has been made the head.

From wives:

> "Now as the church submits to Christ, so also wives should submit to their husbands in everything . . . and the wife must respect her husband." The Greek word translated "submit" is derived from the same word meaning "to yield" in the sense of yielding to another's authority.

According to the Searses:

> Mother-infant attachment is a special bond of closeness between mother and baby. Mother's care enables the young of each species to thrive and, for human babies, to reach their fullest potential. Babies come equipped with behaviors that help mothers deliver the right kind of care. God has placed within mothers both the chemistry and the sensitivity to respond to their babies appropriately. This maternal equipping is what is meant by the phrase "mother's intuition." It helps her get attached to her baby.

Elsewhere the Searses refer to the "science" behind attachment parenting, but the reality is that attachment parenting reflects the Searses' fundamentalist Christian beliefs that traditional gender roles are part of God's plan. The Searses are generally reticent about the religious origins of attachment parenting. They have allowed others to promote the idea that attachment parenting is the way children were raised in prehistoric times and that attachment parenting is supported by science. Neither claim is true.

THE PALEOFANTASY OF ATTACHMENT PARENTING

Just as natural childbirth advocates start with a paleofantasy of birth, imagining that natural childbirth recapitulates it, attachment parenting advocates start with a paleofantasy of parenting. As Charlotte Faircloth explains:

> Typically . . . contemporary foraging societies are used to represent 'natural' patterns of lactation and care. As

stand-ins for earlier hominid hunter-gatherers, statistics concerning length and frequency of lactation are used to demonstrate the ancestral pattern. Local cultural traditions are largely ignored and the !Kung, for example, are treated as passively representative of human biological patterns, existing outside of wider cultural trends and with no culture of their own. The primitive is thus constructed as a site for fantasies of the natural to be played out.[4]

The reality of contemporary indigenous cultures is quite different than attachment parenting advocates imagine. As David F. Lancy, PhD, notes in "Detachment Parenting":

> Anthropologists studying mother-infant relations provide ethnographic descriptions that don't square with the latest orthodoxy. Erchak in rural Liberia describes "Casual nurturance [where Kpelle] mothers carry their babies on their backs and nurse them frequently but do so without really paying much direct attention to them; they continue working or . . . socializing." Paradise records that "When a [Mazahua] mother holds a nursing baby in her arms she frequently has a distracted air and pays almost no attention to the baby." Le Vine observed "Gusii mothers [who] rarely looked at or spoke to their infants and toddlers, even when they were holding and breast-feeding them." In none of these cases did the anthropologists observe any decrement in the mental health of individuals subjected to— in attachment orthodoxy—maternal deprivation.[5]

And we have no idea whether contemporary indigenous cultures bear any resemblance to ancient cultures. Furthermore, the paleofantasy of parenting imagines that hunter-gather societies have no cultures at all, merely living like their nonhominid ancestors. The truth is that hunter-gatherer societies did have cultures and those cultures differed from place to place and changed across the tens of thousands of years of hunter-gatherer society. When we consider how much parenting itself has changed from our parents' generation to ours, it seems absurd to imagine that parenting never changed at all during the many generations of our prehistoric ancestors.

The parenting practices of our hunter-gatherer ancestors did not represent perfect parenting in their own time; there is no reason to think they represent perfect parenting in our time. What are the metrics by which any of this could be judged, anyway?

THE PRINCIPLES OF ATTACHMENT PARENTING

According to Attachment Parenting International, the eight principles of attachment parenting are:

1. **Prepare for Pregnancy, Birth, and Parenting.** . . . [C]hildbirth without the use of interventions shows the best start to the parent-infant bond.
2. **Feed with Love and Respect.** . . . Breastfeeding is the healthiest infant-feeding choice. The physiology of breastfeeding promotes a high degree of maternal responsiveness.
3. **Respond with Sensitivity.** . . . Baby-training systems, such as the commonly referred to "cry it out," are inconsistent with this principle.
4. **Use Nurturing Touch.** Parents who "wear" their babies in a sling or wrap are applying this principle.

5. **Ensure Safe Sleep, Physically and Emotionally.**
Many attachment parents share a room with their
young children. Those who exclusively breastfeed and
who take necessary safety precautions may prefer to
share their bed.

6. **Provide Consistent and Loving Care.** Secure attachment depends on continuity of care by a single primary
caregiver. Ideally, this is the parent.

7. **Practice Positive Discipline.** There is a strong push
against physical punishment in recent years, but
research shows that all forms of punishment, including punitive time-outs, can not only be ineffective in
teaching children boundaries in their behavior but also
harmful to psychological and emotional development.

8. **Strive for Balance in Your Personal and Family Life.**
Attachment Parenting is a family-centered approach in
that all members of the family have equal value.[6]

The phase "research shows" is repeated over and over, yet no
research is provided to substantiate these principles.

As you may have noticed, attachment parenting is highly
labor intensive, particularly for mothers. That's not a coincidence
because, as will be discussed in chapter 10, attachment parenting,
although ostensibly about babies and children, is at its very core
about controlling mothers.

ATTACHMENT PARENTING VERSUS ATTACHMENT THEORY

What do we know about attachment between infants and small
children and their parents?

The scientific field of attachment theory was defined by a

trio of brilliant researchers: John Bowlby, Donald Winnicott, and Harry Harlow. Each studied the minimal requirements for infants and small children to form attachments to a parent or caregiver. To do so, they looked at extreme emotional deprivation.

After World War II, Bowlby worked with children orphaned by the war and subsequently housed in orphanages. The World Health Organization asked him to write a report on the mental health of these children; the report was published in 1951.

> Infants become attached to adults who are sensitive and responsive in social interactions with the infant, and who remain as consistent caregivers for some months during the period from about six months to two years of age.[7]

Winnicott refined attachment theory with his concept of the "good enough" mother:

> [Winnicott] thought that parents did not need to be perfectly attuned, but just "ordinarily devoted" or "good enough" to protect the baby from often experiencing overwhelming extremes of discomfort and distress, emotional or physical.[8]

Harlow also studied extreme deprivation.[9] Many of us have heard of his experiments with baby monkeys and wire "mother" monkeys.

> Dr. Harlow created inanimate surrogate mothers for the rhesus infants from wire and wood. Each infant became attached to its particular mother, recognizing its unique face and preferring it above all others. . . .

[H]e presented the infants with a cloth mother and a wire mother under two conditions. In one situation, the wire mother held a bottle with food and the cloth mother held no food. In the other situation, the cloth mother held the bottle and the wire mother had nothing.

Overwhelmingly, the infant macaques preferred spending their time clinging to the cloth mother. Even when only the wire mother could provide nourishment, the monkeys visited her only to feed. Harlow concluded that there was much more to the mother/infant relationship than milk and that this "contact comfort" was essential to the psychological development and health of infant monkeys and children.

Harlow also looked at monkeys raised in total social isolation:

In the total isolation experiments baby monkeys would be left alone for three, six, 12, or 24 months of "total social deprivation." The experiments produced monkeys that were severely psychologically disturbed. Harlow wrote:

"The effects of 6 months of total social isolation were so devastating and debilitating that we had assumed initially that 12 months of isolation would not produce any additional decrement. This assumption proved to be false; 12 months of isolation almost obliterated the animals socially."[10]

Bowlby, Winnicott, and Harlow elucidated important principles. Simply attending to the bodily needs of infants and children is not enough to ensure health. Infants and small children must be given the opportunity to form an attachment to their caregiver. The caregiver does *not* need to be extraordinarily attuned to the child's needs, merely "good enough."

Attachment parenting, as described by William Sears and others, is supposed to be based on attachment theory, but when you actually compare the two ideas, you will see little connection at all.

THE CONTINGENT NATURE OF ATTACHMENT IN ATTACHMENT PARENTING

Attachment parenting rests on the assumption that maternal-infant attachment is contingent, and in the absence of specific practices, children will end up "detached." Ironically, given that attachment parenting is promoted as "natural," the idea that maternal-infant attachment occurs naturally, that mother and child might love each other simply because they belong to each other, is rejected out of hand. Instead, specific ritualized practices must be employed and mothers must be taught these practices by an army of experts, including parenting gurus, midwives, doulas, and lactation consultants, among others.

As Faircloth notes:

> It hardly seems controversial to say that, today, we have a cultural concern with how "attached" parents are to their children. Midwives encourage mothers to try "skin-to-skin" contact with their babies to improve "bonding" after childbirth, a wealth of experts advocate "natural" parenting styles which encourage "attachment" with infants.

Bill and Martha Sears also problematize mother-infant attachment; it doesn't come naturally but requires expert advice:

> The skills for attachment certainly don't come easily to many women in our culture because we have lost, to a great extent, the benefit of a close-knit society where the young ones can learn by watching the experienced ones. This is the reason why we have books and classes on parenting, and support groups.

If attachment parenting is not based on attachment theory, where did the scientific justification come from? It came not from the study of humans, but of nonprimate animals. Animals like ducklings were shown to imprint on whatever caretaker they saw first during an attachment window. Attachment parenting theorists simply extrapolated from that, insisting that human infants "bonded" to their mothers during an attachment window around birth.

According to Faircloth:

> The argument was that a child's first hours, weeks, and months of life had a lasting impact on the entire course of the child's development. . . . Birth, in particular, was singled out as one of the "critical moments" for bonding to take place. After birth, new mothers were told to look into the eyes of their infant, hold their naked child, preferably with skin-to-skin contact, and breastfeed for optimal bonding. . . .
>
> From the outset, successful bonding thus required . . . a set of behaviours that maintained proximity with one's child.

These behaviors include unmedicated vaginal birth, breast-feeding, baby wearing (carrying the baby against the mother's body using a cloth sling), and infant co-sleeping. Yet everything we know about infant attachment tells us none of those elements is required for secure infant attachment. Indeed, attachment of the infant to the mother (or other primary caregiver) is virtually guaranteed in all but the most extreme cases of abuse and neglect. Moreover, there is nothing in attachment theory that suggests that attachment security can be increased or needs to be increased above the attachment that all infants and children will naturally form with their caregivers.

Attachment parenting is in fact an incorrect appropriation of attachment theory. Attachment theory tells us that all that is necessary for secure attachment is a "good enough" mother. Attachment parenting warns that anything less than a perfect mother poses a risk to secure attachment and thus to a child's well-being.

FETISHIZING PROXIMITY

In *The Attachment Parenting Book*, Bill and Martha Sears proclaim:

> Where does a baby belong? We believe that most of the time, young babies should be in the arms of their parents, wherever their parents may be. That's why we've become great advocates of the baby sling, a simple cloth baby carrier that holds an infant close to Mother or Father's body. You use the sling when you go out, and you use it around the house as well. It's like wearing your baby—which is why we call this parenting style babywearing.

The beauty of babywearing is that you are, literally, attached.[11]

According to Attachment Parenting International:

> Attachment Parenting has been studied extensively for over 60 years by psychology and child development researchers, and more recently, by researchers studying the brain. These studies revealed that infants are born "hardwired" with strong needs to be nurtured and to remain physically close to the primary caregiver, usually the mother, during the first few years of life. The child's emotional, physical, and neurological development is greatly enhanced when these basic needs are met consistently and appropriately. These needs can be summarized as *proximity, protection, and predictability*.[12]

Actually, there has been no research demonstrating that constant close physical proximity is needed for mother-infant bonding. Attachment parenting reduces the long, complex, and emotionally fraught journey of parenting to physical proximity between a mother and her infant. Supposedly, the essence of parenting is literally binding your baby to yourself with baby wearing, breastfeeding, and co-sleeping. In attachment parenting, the word attachment has a dual function. The AP mother proclaims her stronger emotional attachment to her child by literally attaching the child to her body.

As Rebecca Kukla, a feminist philosopher writing about fetishizing proximity in her book *Mass Hysteria: Motherhood, Culture and Mother's Bodies*,[13] confirms, the insistence on proximity reflects moral values, not scientific evidence.

> [T]he relationship between mother and child is figured spatially, in terms of material proximity and nearness, and as a continuation of the material bond of the umbilical cord. This proximity is figured as both natural and appropriate. This relationship of . . . proximity between the infant and the maternal body continues to be positioned as the source and symbol of more abstract, appropriate moral and social relations.

The alternate name for attachment parenting, intensive mothering, is particularly revealing. First, attachment parenting devolves almost exclusively on mothers. It isn't a parenting practice so much as it is a mothering practice. Second, intensive mothering reflects the true focus of attachment parenting; it isn't about what children need as much as it is about how mothers should behave.

ATTACHMENT PARENTING AND PARENTING IN NATURE

The phrase "it takes a village to raise a child" comes from indigenous societies. In attachment parenting, ironically, it takes only a mother following a rigid set of behaviors that in truth have little or nothing to do with raising healthy, well-adjusted children.

In nature the burden of child-rearing is shared with grandmothers and older siblings. Indeed, some researchers believe that menopause confers an evolutionary advantage for humans because women who can no longer bear children turn to nurturing their grandchildren, thus providing their children with significant benefits. Parenting in nature involves being nurtured and educated by an extended kin group.

Eve reflects on the consequences of her slavish devotion to attachment parenting:

> *I adhered with near religious fervor to the attachment parent dogma of always being within arm's reach of my nursing baby . . . and had small feelings of quasi contempt for my sisters-in-law. They were giving formula and pumping/storing milk so that they could leave their babies with Grandma and Grandpa (my parents) and enjoy dates and weekend getaways with their husbands. . . .*
>
> *My wonderful loving parents were so much closer and affectionate with my brother's children because I was the idiot who denied my parents overnight fun with the babies. My children missed out on inside jokes, running gags, and playful familiarity with my parents because I wanted to be the best, most preindustrialized style mother.*
>
> *I felt the full error of my ways when my dad died and my nieces and nephews cried and shared tales of "remember the time when we slept at Poppie's house and he . . ." I had denied my children the loving influence of my parents because I was too busy being an attachment parent.*

Ironically, many of the practices associated with contemporary attachment parenting didn't even exist in nature. Tandem nursing (simultaneously nursing an infant and a toddler), one of the hallmarks of attachment parenting, doesn't exist in the animal world or in indigenous societies. When the next offspring is born, breast milk is reserved exclusively for the nurturing of that infant and the older offspring is not allowed to continue nursing.

Traditionally, baby wearing is not designed for emotional closeness; it is designed to protect babies from predators while mothers work around or outside the home. Indeed, the need for women to work, both around and outside the home, is integral to the survival of the group in hunter-gatherer societies. Similarly, the family bed was a reflection of the need for group protection, and later on a reflection of economic realities when families were lucky to have a single bed, not a focus of nurturing.

If our hunter-gatherer ancestors could reach across the centuries to give parenting advice, they would likely tell us that it takes a village to raise a child, not a MOBY Wrap baby-wearing sling.

DOES ATTACHMENT PARENTING LEAD TO MATERNAL DEPRESSION?

At a dinner party several years ago, one of the guests, a psychiatric social worker, asked me what I do. I explained that I blog about issues of pseudoscience in parenting. She became very excited and asked me if I had ever heard of attachment parenting. She had been seeing an increasing number of young mothers with depression and related issues. In her experience, the increase in young mothers with depression is related to the rise of attachment parenting that appears to dramatically increase social isolation, stress, and feelings of failure.

She's not the only one to observe this phenomenon. "Insight into the Parenthood Paradox: Mental Health Outcomes of Intensive Mothering"[14] by Kathryn Rizzo and colleagues was designed to collect quantitative data on the relationship between intensive parenting and maternal mental health outcomes including stress, depression, and life satisfaction. The authors hypothesized that intensive parenting attitudes would result in greater levels of stress and depression and lower levels of life satisfaction.

They found that the belief that mothers are the most capable

parent was associated with higher levels of stress and lower levels
of life satisfaction.

> In prior research, mothers have expressed difficulty
> selecting an alternate caregiver because they felt that no
> one else, including the child's father, could provide the
> same degree of love, commitment, and skill. If women
> believe they are the most capable caregiver, they may
> limit help from others, a practice known as maternal
> gatekeeping. This may account for the lower levels of
> social support reported by women who endorsed [these]
> attitudes.

The belief that parenting is difficult was also related to higher
levels of depression and stress, as well as lower levels of life satisfaction. The same held true for the belief that parents' lives should
revolve around their children.

> [W]hen women feel they must subsume their needs to
> the needs of their child, they lose a sense of personal
> freedom, which may result in women experiencing
> negative mental health outcomes (e.g., lower levels of
> life satisfaction).

The authors note that the "results of this study suggest that the
negative maternal mental health outcomes associated with parenting may be accounted for by women's endorsement of intensive
parenting attitudes."

If intensive mothering is related to so many negative mental
health outcomes, why do women do it? They may think that it
makes them better mothers, so they are willing to sacrifice their
own mental health to enhance their children's cognitive and socio-

emotional outcomes. However, given that a considerable body of research indicates that the children of women with poor mental health (e.g., depression) are at higher risk for negative outcomes, intensive parenting may have the opposite effect on children from what parents intend.

ATTACHMENT PARENTING AND POSTPARTUM DEPRESSION

In a piece entitled "Do Ideal Images of Motherhood Impact Post-partum Depression?" journalist Avital Norman Nathman writes:

> The period of time immediately after having a baby—especially if he or she is your first—can be an incredibly fragile one. . . . It can be even more challenging when faced with images of "ideal" motherhood everywhere you turn.[15]

She speaks with an expert, Dr. Jessica Zucker, a clinical psychologist specializing in women's reproductive and maternal mental health:

> "Cultural ideals surrounding motherhood serve to stimulate shame and secrecy when it comes to postpartum challenges," Dr. Zucker told me. "As a result of media's portrayal of idyllic early motherhood, women who don't fit perfectly into this ubiquitous image often report feeling like 'failures' and take their troubles underground."

But these ideals don't come from the media; they come from attachment parenting, including claims such as:

< Women who have pharmacologic pain relief in labor have "given in" and put their own needs above the "risk of exposing their babies to drugs."

< Women who have C-sections have "failed" at birth.

< Women who have pain relief can't bond to their babies.

< Women who don't have enough breast milk are either failures or liars, since "every woman has enough breast milk."

< Women must have their babies in close physical proximity to them at all times and never have a break.

< Women should not allow their partners, mothers, mothers-in-law, or babysitters to bear any part of the burden of child care.

As Norman Nathman points out, such idealized representations have the power to harm fragile new mothers. Who would be so cruel as to promote these accusations to a new mother? Not anyone who cared about women's mental health.

Norman Nathman writes about potential solutions to this problem of maternal anguish:

> One way to help combat this range of detrimental representation is to provide safe spaces for mothers to talk without judgment. . . .
>
> Another solution is to provide a much more varied and diverse picture of what motherhood truly is about.

I agree! When are attachment parenting advocates going to realize that their failure to provide a much more varied and diverse picture of what good motherhood is truly about is harming women?

THE TRUTH ABOUT ATTACHMENT PARENTING

From the cover of *Time* magazine[16] ("Are You Mom Enough?") to the playgrounds to social media and the Internet, we are busily judging other mothers and how they comport with the ideology of attachment parenting.

Who profits from such a paradigm? Who pays the price? Who is excluded from the practice and who avoids responsibility altogether? These are the questions that are worth examining.

Who Profits?

According to a recent position paper, "Governing Motherhood: Who Pays and Who Profits?,"[17] written by Phyllis Rippeyoung and published by the Canadian Centre for Policy Alternatives, the profit is restricted to self-proclaimed parenting "experts" like Dr. William Sears and his acolytes.

Who Pays?

Mothers pay . . . in a myriad of ways including lost earnings and lost time for themselves and increased feelings of guilt.

Attachment parenting is a philosophy of privilege. It is completely inaccessible to women who are poor, work at low-wage menial jobs, and lack the support of a partner who earns enough to make attachment parenting financially feasible. Now, in addition to struggling to provide their children with the basic necessities of living, these women are denigrated for being unable to provide their children with what has been deemed requisite emotional support.

Who's Excluded?

Fathers are excluded.

Despite its name, attachment parenting renders fathers peripheral in the exact same way as the oft-mocked lifestyle choices of the 1950s. The father exists to provide financial support; the mother exists to provide her presence, her labor, and her emotional support.

Who Avoids Responsibility Altogether?

The only role for government imagined by many attachment parenting proponents is to pressure women into practicing the tenets of attachment parenting or, at the very least, shame them for not doing so by aggressively promoting breastfeeding and other treasured imperatives of attachment parenting.

As Rippeyoung notes in specific regard to breastfeeding:

> This individualizing of responsibility for child welfare has also been seen among breastfeeding proponents, as most explicitly illustrated in an editorial by Dr. Ruth Lawrence, a founder of the Academy of Breastfeeding Medicine. In her essay "The Elimination of Poverty One Child at a Time," she argues that breastfeeding is the panacea for health and cognitive inequalities between poor and non-poor children. She ends the piece by writing that breastfeeding may be the only gift that poor mothers have to offer their children.
>
> Although neglectful and abusive parenting has been shown to explain multiple forms of inequalities in child outcomes, I have been unable to find any research assessing whether breastfeeding, baby-sling wearing,

co-sleeping, or the other attachment parenting practices advocated by the Sears Family or others will actually reduce either poverty or the consequences of growing up poor, one child at a time or otherwise.

The author concludes:

If policy makers are truly interested in improving child health and welfare, more needs to be done to address the problems faced by families comprehensively and structurally; not only in terms of training individual mothers to behave in particular, culturally defined ways.

I couldn't agree more.

NATURAL PARENTING TREATS CHILDREN LIKE PRODUCTS, NOT PEOPLE

An additional problem with natural parenting (natural childbirth, lactivism, and attachment parenting), besides the fact that it is not supported by science, is that it is deterministic.

At its heart, natural parenting views a child as an object to be acted upon to create the desired result, an adult with specific middle- to upper-middle-class achievements: smart, talented, and ready to enter the economic competition of adulthood at a high level. What's particularly striking about natural parenting is not merely that parents wish to raise children they can brag about, but that they think they have the recipe to do it.

This deterministic view of parenting has important implications for children, parents, and social policy.

Consider breastfeeding. This is a paradigmatic case of natural parenting beliefs being turned into public policy. When and why did the government think it should get involved in promoting breastfeeding, which as discussed has been shown in first world countries to have only trivial benefits? There's not much question that the government has inserted itself into breastfeeding promotion at the behest of lactivists, despite the fact that there couldn't be a more intimate, fundamental personal choice than how women use their own breasts.

Lactivism, like all of natural parenting, is a one-size-fits-all policy. The fundamental assumptions of lactivism is that *all* children will do "better" if breastfed, that *all* women make enough breast milk to satisfy the needs of *all* infants, that *every* child's brain is "improved" by breastfeeding, and that *all* women should be more concerned with using their breasts to feed babies than with using their minds and talents to work outside the home and meet any of their own needs. Those assumptions are sweeping and false.

The more important issue, though, is what breastfeeding policy tells us about the way we conceptualize children. We don't see them as people, unique individuals with unique needs. We see them as future adults, poised to become the adults we desire *if only* the parents fill them with the correct inputs. But any parent who has more than one child knows that the parenting strategies that make one child happy may be utterly wrong for another child who has the same parents, in the same family, growing up under the same economic and sociocultural conditions.

The implications of the determinism of natural parenting are enormous. The message that natural parenting sends, particularly to mothers, is "It's all up to you," and if things don't work out, "It's all your fault."

But parenting is *not* deterministic. Parents can't create perfect adults no matter how desperately they wish they could. And good parents can, with the best effort and intentions, raise children who are average or below average, emotionally fragile, subject to the perils of addiction, or even criminals.

Fortunately, most children are resilient. If they were not, I would fear we are raising a generation that will struggle because we ignore who children *are*—their needs, desires, dreams, talents, and limitations—in favor of the adults that parents desire their children to *become*.

NATURAL PARENTING'S BIG LIE

"Motherhood, Screened Off"[18] by Susan Dominus recently appeared in *The New York Times*. Ostensibly this is a piece about pushing aside technology to reconnect with our children. Dominus suggests that our use of technology has rendered previously transparent adult actions opaque to children and that is a problem.

> When my mother was curious about the weather, I saw her pick up the front page of the newspaper and scan for the information. The same, of course, could be said of how she apprised herself of the news. I always knew to whom she was talking because, before caller ID, all conversations started with what now seems like elaborate explicitness ("Hi, Toby, this is Flora").

I took something different away from the piece. I read it as an example of our contemporary obsession with artisanal (i.e., natural) parenting, the belief that our children are products that are rendered "high quality" by small-batch production using traditional labor-intensive methods. Any moment spent not nurturing, teaching, or connecting with our children (for example, looking at weather.com on your iPhone) is a moment wasted.

Simply put, if you aren't suffering, you must be doing mothering wrong.

In the world of natural parenting, traditional and traditionally painful and inconvenient processes are required to produce perfect children. The mother takes no shortcuts and avoids all conveniences, thereby producing superior children. Greater suffering equals higher quality. Unmedicated childbirth is therefore "better," since it is a traditional method involving lots of maternal suffering. Breastfeeding is supposedly "best," since it involves maternal time, effort, discomfort, and inconvenience. Attachment parenting (baby wearing, family bed, no sleep training) is purportedly better because every moment of every mother's day should involve her child.

Adult activities must be transparent to children—hence the author's lament that her children don't know what she is doing when she is using her phone. Adult activities must be justifiable to children—hence the author's worry that although she is physically at their soccer practice (where she is not needed and presumably not a focus of their concern), they might look up and see her on her phone and won't realize that she is engaged in something meaningful (reading literature) rather than performing tasks or amusing herself.

> I have started to narrate my use of the phone when I am around my kids. "I'm emailing your teacher back," I tell them, or, "I'm now sending that text you asked me to send about that sleepover," in the hopes that I can defang the device's bad reputation, its inherent whiff of self-absorption.

What's the real problem with a little maternal self-absorption? It means the mother is not suffering enough!

My husband thinks no amount of narration will change the way our kids feel about the phone. The problem, he says, is that whenever I grab it, they know that I am also holding a portal, as magical as the one in Narnia's wardrobe and with the same potential to transport me to another world or to infinite worlds. . . . Perhaps they sense how vast the reach of the device is and how little they know of what that vastness contains; at any moment, the size of the gap between them and me is unknowable.

And it's wrong for nine-year-old children to be deprived of their mother's rapt attention for an unknowable amount of minutes, because . . . why?

It means the mother is not giving enough of herself!

The ultimate irony of contemporary natural parenting is that what is imagined as the "way things were" before technology could not be further from the truth. When mothers had less technology at their disposal, they had *less* time for nurturing, teaching, or connecting with their children. And here's the kicker: they weren't worried about nurturing, teaching, or connecting with their children on a moment-by-moment basis; they were too busy simply trying to survive.

Prior to the advent of technology, children spent *more* time outside the direct purview of their mothers. They went outdoors for hours at a time to play with other children. They did chores (real chores, not just making their beds) necessary to the family's existence; in other words, they worked for their keep.

The truth is that children are not artisanal products whose quality is proportional to the time their mother spent nurturing them while ignoring her own needs. They do not require the caress of the maternal gaze every waking moment of their lives.

They do not need constant maternal interaction; indeed, they can be *stifled* from constant maternal interaction.

What children need is knowledge of their mother's love and concern; her suffering merely reflects our conceit that children are our products and by suffering we can make them what we want them to be.

ATTACHMENT PARENTING: 50 SHADES OF BLACK OR WHITE

If there's anything I've learned in nearly thirty years of parenting, it's that different children, even from the same family, need different things. And if there's anything I've learned from practicing medicine, it's that there are many different ways (cultural traditions, religious traditions, family traditions) to raise children successfully.

But not for attachment parents, for whom there is only one way—their way.

I'm reminded of the famous quote from Henry Ford, describing the sale of the Model T: "Any customer can have a car painted any color that he wants so long as it is black."

In the world of attachment parenting, a mother can have any birth she wants, so long as it is vaginal, unmedicated, and "unhindered."

A mother can feed a baby in whatever way she prefers, so long as it is breastfeeding.

A mother can carry her child any way she wants, so long as it is strapped to her body, not in a stroller or, heaven forfend, not carried or placed in an enclosed play space.

In other words, in attachment parenting, there are 50 shades, but all of them are black or white, bad or good. Attachment parents don't do nuance.

Epidurals bad. Natural childbirth good. Never mind that most women experience agonizing pain.

Cesarean bad. Vaginal birth good. Never mind that there are countless situations in which a C-section is the better, safer mode of birth for both baby and mother.

Bottle-feeding bad. Breastfeeding good. Never mind that there are women who can't make enough milk, find breastfeeding too painful, or simply prefer bottle-feeding.

Cribs bad. Family bed good.

All parenting choices can be characterized as bad or good, nothing in between. There is absolutely no appreciation for the concept that what is good for one mother-child pair may need to be modified slightly or dramatically in order to be best for another mother-child pair. There is absolutely no appreciation that when it comes to parenting, there are infinite shades of all colors because there are infinite combinations of mother and child.

Why are parenting choices black or white in the world of attachment parenting? Because attachment parenting has nothing to do with parenting and nothing to do with children. It's all about women and how they view themselves in relation to other women. There's only black (not a good mother like me) and white (mirroring my own choices back to me).

But real parenting is about trying to meet the varied needs of many family members, within varied cultural and religious traditions, not to mention a multitude of specific family dynamics. In the real world, there is no magic recipe for raising healthy, happy children.

In other words, in the real world of parenting, there are endless shades of every color, not simply black and white.

PART II

THE NATURAL PARENTING INDUSTRY

Who Hijacked Childbirth?

There have always been midwives. Ever since our ancestors acquired the ability to walk upright, human childbirth has been fraught with extreme risk to both mother and baby. The first midwives were those who recognized that assistance in childbirth can minimize those risks. They understood that something as simple as massaging a woman's uterus after childbirth could prevent life-threatening hemorrhage, and that different fetal positions like breech posed specific problems that could be overcome with specific maneuvers. Over time, they acquired knowledge of the medicinal properties of certain plants and gave extracts to women with the intention of starting labor or stopping bleeding.

Above all, ancient midwives were rationalists. Their very existence was predicated on the inherent dangers of childbirth, and everything they did was devoted to keeping women and babies safe. They supplemented magic incantations with empirical observation. They noted what worked and what did not, and they faithfully strove to incorporate those scientific observations into practice. Midwives, in other words, were the obstetricians of old.

Despite profound changes in the human condition, midwifery changed very little. Midwifery knowledge grew, of course, and that knowledge was supplemented by appeals to whatever forces were deemed to be in charge at the time (nature, gods, the church), but the purpose always remained the same. And the faithful adherence to rationalism (as opposed to the often outlandish theories held by doctors up to the nineteenth century) ensured that midwives provided the best possible care to the women they served.

That was certainly what I understood midwifery to be when I entered medical school, and that view was then reinforced by working extensively with certified nurse-midwives in the hospital setting. I found them to be highly educated, very experienced, and capable of providing a more personalized form of care for laboring mothers. But in recent years, especially since the 1980s and 1990s, midwifery has changed into something very different.

In fact, I think it is fair to say that midwifery has been hijacked by radicals.

THE NATURAL CHILDBIRTH INDUSTRY

For most of human existence, childbirth was the painful, dangerous, but unavoidable way to have a child. Over the past fifty years, in first world countries, the view of a birth that both mother and child survived has been transformed from a cause for thanksgiving into a virtually guaranteed, totally expected outcome. As a result, a space was created for the rise of a new industry that focuses on childbirth, not as a way to have a child, but as a way to have an experience.

Women often have an aha moment when they realize that natural childbirth is an industry, complete with trade unions, professional organizations, and grassroots activists. Many people profit from the natural childbirth industry, and therefore lobby aggressively on its behalf among state and national legislatures. Natural childbirth is big business.

How big?

Until the twentieth century, midwifery required no formal education, just a period of apprenticeship. With the rise of modern obstetrics, midwives saw the need to professionalize in order to compete and, emulating European nurse-midwives, created the credential of certified nurse-midwife (CNM). These were nurses who had undergone additional training in midwifery.

The first two schools of nurse-midwifery were opened in the 1930s, but it was not until the 1970s that the profession began to experience a resurgence. Midwifery grew from 275 CNMs in 1963 to more than 4,000 in 1995 to over 11,000 today.[1]

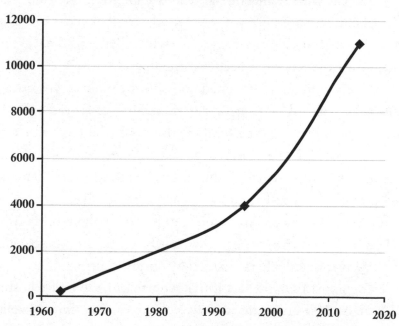

Certified Nurse Midwives

The proportion of births attended by midwives has also risen from 3 percent in 1989 to 8.2 percent of births in 2013 (12 percent of vaginal births in that year).[2] Midwifery salaries are substantial, averaging from $75,000 to $99,000 across most of the country.[3] Doulas and childbirth educators have made similar gains.

Why do even sophisticated people fail to recognize that natural childbirth is an industry? It's probably because they equate "industry" with large amounts of money. True, individual professional natural childbirth advocates don't make a lot of money, but for most, it represents 100 percent of their income. That's why they have a tremendous financial incentive to convince you to buy their products and services.

That doesn't mean that those who promote natural childbirth don't believe in it. Its advocates believe fiercely in what they promote and sell—normal birth as the holy grail of childbirth, midwives as the guardians of normal birth, and distrust of obstetricians, whom they correctly identify as their chief competition.

The next two chapters detail the rise and dominance of the natural childbirth industry, the very industry that seeks to make the experience of having a baby a lifestyle choice, and the ways in which the experience has been commodified.

Modern midwifery was made possible by modern obstetrics, which has ushered in an age when childbirth *seems* safe. Previously doctors were called to childbirth in only the most dire circumstances. With the switch to routine hospitalization for birth and the routine presence of obstetricians and, in particular, the easy access to pain relief, midwifery went into decline.

Obstetricians were only too happy to supplant midwives. While midwives themselves make much of this economic competition, blaming deliberate action by obstetricians in an attempt to stifle competition, the fact is that women came to prefer hospital birth because of its safety and increased comfort. So midwives fought back by deriding what obstetricians offered and offering the exact opposite.

< If obstetricians medicalized childbirth to make it safer, then midwives would demedicalize it to make it more enjoyable, and for added impact, would declare that childbirth was safe *before* obstetricians got involved.

< If obstetricians offered screening tests and measures to prevent complications, then midwives would insist that "trusting birth" was all that was needed.

< If obstetricians offered pain relief, midwives would proclaim that feeling the pain improved the experience, tested one's mettle, and made childbirth safer.

< If obstetricians whisked babies off to pediatricians to make sure that they were healthy, midwives would claim that skin-to-skin contact between mother and infant in the first moments after birth was crucial to creating a lifelong bond.

< If obstetricians insisted that modern obstetrics was based on science, midwives would accuse them of ignoring science, and if that didn't stick, midwives would insist that scientific evidence was not the only form of knowledge.

< If obstetricians placed the highest value on a healthy mother and a healthy baby, midwives would place the highest value on a fulfilling birth experience.

No matter what obstetricians offered, midwives would insist that it was unnecessary, disempowering, harmful, and contradicted by the scientific evidence. Midwives would wrest childbirth back from paternalistic doctors and give it to those to whom they believed it rightly belonged—the midwives themselves. And the entire project would be promoted as being in the best interests of women and babies.

This has been noted by feminist theorists. Ellen Annandale and Judith Clark, authors of the widely quoted paper "What Is Gender? Feminist Theory and the Sociology of Human Reproduction,"[4] describe contemporary midwifery as

> the largely unresearched antithesis of obstetrics. An alternative is called into existence in powerful and convincing terms, while at the same time its central precepts (such as "women controlled," "natural birth") are vaguely drawn and in practical terms carry little meaning.

The effort by midwives to reclaim what they considered to be their "turf" has been a multistage process involving

- the denial of the inherent dangers of childbirth
- criticism by sociologists and anthropologists of the medicalization of childbirth
- creation of an alternative world of internal legitimacy to transmit the "findings" of midwifery research
- an insistence that obstetricians don't follow the scientific evidence
- the elevation of process over outcome/experience over safety
- the elevation of normal birth as the holy grail of childbirth
- the proclamation of themselves as guardians of normal birth
- ultimately, the "commodification" of the birth experience

In the process, midwives and their associated paraprofessionals, doulas and childbirth educators, have become radicalized.

DENIAL OF THE INHERENT DANGERS OF CHILDBIRTH

In chapter 1 we saw just how far the philosophy of natural child-birth has strayed from the reality of childbirth prior to modern obstetrics. Childbirth is and has always been, in every time, place, and culture, a dangerous endeavor for mothers and their babies. In industrialized countries in the twenty-first century, the birth of a healthy baby to a healthy mother has become so commonplace that it is taken for granted by natural childbirth advocates. Only someone who has no idea of the medical and historical reality of childbirth could recommend "trusting" birth.

So the entire foundational premise of the philosophy of natu-ral childbirth, that a healthy mother and baby are the natural and nearly inevitable result of birth, is completely false. Everything else in contemporary midwifery and natural childbirth advocacy flows from this spectacular error. Denial of the inherent dangers of childbirth is the keystone of the philosophy of natural child-birth. Without it, the philosophy would collapse.

Complaints about the medicalization of childbirth reflect this profound misunderstanding. No one complains about the medi-calization of brain surgery or the medicalization of the treatment of gunshot wounds or snakebites. That's because everyone under-stands that in the absence of medicalization of brain surgery or treatment of gunshot wounds or snakebites, people will die.

It is also not a coincidence that complaints about the medi-calization of childbirth come primarily from people who are not trained in obstetrics, such as anthropologists and sociologists. While anthropologists and sociologists can provide valuable criticism of cultural mores, their critique of modern obstetrics is deeply flawed by their failure to understand that death and dis-ability in childbirth is not a cultural concern, but a factual one.

WHO RADICALIZED MIDWIFERY?

As discussed at the beginning of this chapter, midwifery changed very little across the centuries. Midwives were the obstetricians of the past, focusing on outcomes and not the birth experience.

The improved safety of birth created both a problem and an opportunity for midwives. The problem was that obstetricians could promise safer outcomes. The opportunity was the chance to now emphasize the quality of the birth experience. This privileging of process over outcome was an outgrowth of feminist theory.

Many of the early midwifery theorists were difference feminists, women who moved from insisting that women are equal to men (and therefore have the same rights) to insisting that women are different from men and that those differences should be valued. Among the difference feminists were two types of radical feminists who have profoundly changed the way that childbirth is understood. These two groups of feminists are biological essentialists and feminist anti-rationalists.

Broadly speaking, the biological essentialists are characterized by a belief that women are defined by their biology and that their biological differences from men should be celebrated. The premier biological essentialist in the natural childbirth movement is Sheila Kitzinger.[5] The anti-rationalists are essentialists but with a twist. While rationalists view reason as the ultimate source of human knowledge, anti-rationalism privileges intuition and spiritual beliefs. In the view of a feminist anti-rationalist, reasoning is the preserve of men, and women have "different ways of knowing." The premier anti-rationalist theorist in the childbirth movement is Robbie Davis-Floyd.[6]

The essentialists and the anti-rationalists in the natural childbirth arena share quite a few characteristics. Almost exclusively Western white women of the privileged classes, they believe that they speak for all women because all women purportedly have the same needs and desires. They simply assume that they represent non-Western women and women of color. Many are sociologists and anthropologists. Curiously, although they have little or no practical knowledge of childbirth or modern obstetrics, they don't view that lack of knowledge to be a problem.

You can recognize them by what they say. The biological essentialists are fond of catchphrases like "trust birth" and "pregnancy is not a disease." They insist that obstetrics has "pathologized" childbirth and can display a shocking and callous fatalism by dismissing infant deaths with the dictum that "some babies are not meant to live."

The anti-rationalists in the childbirth arena are distinguished, not surprisingly, by their rejection of reason as the source of knowledge. They dismiss science as a male form of "authoritative knowledge" on the understanding that there are "other ways of knowing," such as intuition. Many are postmodernists who believe that reality is radically subjective, that rationality is unnecessary, and that "including the nonrational is sensible midwifery."

The difference between biological essentialists and anti-rationalists is, not surprisingly, in their view of rationalism. Henci Goer can be counted among the true biological essentialists.[7] The biological essentialists are represented by organizations such as Lamaze and the American College of Nurse-Midwives (ACNM). They worship the "natural" on the assumption that biology determines what is best for all women. Nonetheless, they believe that science is nongendered and valuable, the standard by which claims about childbirth should be judged. They freely quote scientific papers and insist that their views of childbirth are "evidence based," even when these views are clearly not. They still value empirical knowledge and advanced education, despite their constant misrepresentation.

The anti-rationalists reject science as male, and unfairly regarded as authoritative merely because it is male. To the extent that science supports their claims, they are willing to brandish scientific papers as "proof," but they explicitly reject rationalism when it does not accord with their personal beliefs, feelings, and opinions. They do not value empirical knowledge and reject rigorous education.

The grandmother of anti-rationalism among childbirth advocates is Ina May Gaskin,[8] and the Midwives Alliance of North America (MANA), which is in part her creation, is the primary American organizational exponent of anti-rationalism in childbirth. Radical midwifery theorists like the aforementioned British midwife Soo Downe and Australian midwife Jenny Parratt provide the ideological underpinnings of anti-rationalism within midwifery.

These midwives insist that intuition and spiritual beliefs are as important as or more important than science. They are convinced that trusting birth and fighting fear are more efficacious in preventing complications than scientific tests and fetal monitoring. They make claims such as "the safest place to give birth is where the mother feels safest."

A paper entitled "Including the Nonrational Is Sensible Midwifery"[9] offers some of the best examples of anti-rationalist midwifery beliefs.

> [W]hen . . . bleeding begins unexpectedly, the expert midwife will respond with either or both rational and nonrational ways of thinking. Depending upon all the particularities of the situation the midwife may focus on supporting love between the woman and her baby; she may call the woman back to her body; and/or she may change to active management of third stage. It is

sensible practice to respond to in-the-moment clinical situations in this way.

Obstetricians, of course, respond to postpartum bleeding with detailed protocols prescribing specific medications a specific course of action. Anti-rationalist midwives disagree:

> Imposing a pre-agreed standard care protocol is irrational because protocols do not allow for optimal clinical decision-making, which requires that we consider all relevant variables prior to making a decision. In our view all relevant variables include nonrational matters of soul and spirit.

Anti-rationalist midwifery places the midwife and her feelings at the center of practice:

> Being open to the nonrational in midwifery practice makes room for midwives to self-reflexively acknowledge aspects of themselves, such as their fears, in a way that does not interfere with their practice. During birth, making room for the nonrational broadens both midwives' and women's knowledge about trust, courage and their own intuitive abilities including the changing capabilities of bodies. And by including the nonrational midwives can then most honestly be with the woman's own fears as she opens her embodied self to her own unique process of childbearing.

Ultimately, the natural childbirth movement, upon close examination, reveals itself to be built upon philosophy that a majority of women would reject. Most women no longer accept that they are supposed to be defined and determined by their biology. Most women believe in the power of science and the safety that following scientific protocol ensures. But natural childbirth advocates do a wonderful job of blurring the roots of their philosophies so that few really get to see them, and therefore most are swayed by the persuasive emotional and financial power they hold instead.

THE SOCIOLOGY/ANTHROPOLOGY OF OBSTETRICS

The chief justification for the radicalization of midwifery comes not from science, but from social science. Midwives and their allies within the disciplines of sociology and anthropology created a narrative claiming that modern obstetrics had nothing to do with science and everything to do with paternalism and greed.

Robbie Davis-Floyd articulates the belief, shared by many midwives, that modern obstetrics was created by men for the benefit and profit of men:

> The demise of the midwife and the rise of the male-attended, mechanically manipulated birth followed close on the heels of the wide cultural acceptance of the metaphor of the body-as-machine in the West, and the accompanying acceptance of the metaphor of the female body as a defective machine—a metaphor that eventually formed the philosophical foundation of modern obstetrics. Obstetrics was thus enjoined by its own conceptual origins to develop tools and technologies for the manipulation and improvement of the inherently defective and therefore anomalous and dangerous process of birth. . . .

The rising science of obstetrics ultimately accomplished this goal by adopting the model of the assembly-line production of goods—the template by which most of the technological wonders of modern society were being produced—as its base metaphor for hospital birth. In accordance with this metaphor, a woman's reproductive tract is treated like a birthing machine by skilled technicians working under semi-flexible timetables to meet production and quality control demands.[10]

Davis-Floyd has managed to cram into just two short paragraphs a host of mistruths, half-truths, and outright lies about modern obstetrics. Tellingly, Davis-Floyd purports to explain the rise of modern obstetrics in opposition to midwifery.

The first lie is one of omission. By omitting the most salient fact about childbirth, that it is and has always been in every time, place, and culture a leading cause of the death of young women and *the* leading cause of death of babies, Davis-Floyd has implied that there was never any need for modern obstetrics in the first place. She insinuates that its raison d'être was malign, to profit from unnecessary interventions, when its entire reason for being is beneficent, to save the lives of mothers and babies and to minimize the pain of childbirth.

Obstetrics and obstetricians are cast in brutal terms, viewing the female body as defective machines, creating assembly lines for the delivery of babies and casting safety as "quality control demands." This, in my view, is abject nonsense, completely divorced from the reality of the practice of obstetrics. It could only be conjured by someone who has no idea of either the history or the medical reality of childbirth.

But instead of acknowledging the fact that it was *women* who came to prefer obstetricians and hospitals over midwives and homebirth, Davis-Floyd spins the more comfortable fiction that obstetricians stole childbirth from midwives by fabricating lies about its dangers. This isn't just insulting to obstetricians; it is also insulting to women, implying as it does that they were not smart enough to see through the manipulative tactics of obstetricians.

It also cast light on one of the favored marketing tactics of the natural childbirth industry, the fantasy that those who reject modern obstetrics are more "educated" than those who practice it. That's why someone like Henci Goer, a layperson with no training in obstetrics, midwifery, and nursing, can claim with a straight face that obstetricians don't follow scientific evidence. It also explains why natural childbirth advocates preen that they have "done their research," when in reality all they have done is imbibe propaganda and research the work of others who echo their own beliefs back to them.

OBSTETRICIANS DON'T FOLLOW THE SCIENTIFIC EVIDENCE?

When natural childbirth advocates leave the echo chamber of their books, conferences, blogs, and message boards, they are often shocked that their assertions about childbirth are greeted with disbelief and even contempt by mainstream medical practitioners. Instead of responding to the disbelief by questioning their own maxims, they just question the legitimacy of obstetricians.

In her book *The Thinking Woman's Guide to a Better Birth*, Henci Goer declares:

> Obstetric practice does not reflect the research evidence because obstetricians actually base their practices on a set of predetermined beliefs. If you start from this

premise, everything about obstetrics, including the inconsistencies between research and practice, makes sense.[11]

Goer insists that obstetricians (with eight years of higher education, extensive study of science and statistics, and four additional years of hands-on experience caring for pregnant women), the people who actually *do* the research that represents the body of scientific evidence, are ignoring their own findings, while midwives and natural childbirth advocates, the people who rarely, if ever, do quantitative scientific research, are assiduously scouring the scientific literature, reading the main obstetric journals each month, and changing their recommendations and practice based on the latest scientific evidence.

That makes no sense at all.

It's an effort to deal with the cognitive dissonance that comes from realizing that obstetricians reject most of the factual claims of natural childbirth advocates. Somebody has to be wrong, and as far as natural childbirth advocates are concerned, it can't be them. After all, all of those in the natural childbirth community—including the speakers at conferences, the authors of books, and the editors of journals—agree with one another. So if the obstetricians disagree, they must be ignoring what everyone in the natural childbirth community *knows* to be true.

HOW NATURAL CHILDBIRTH ADVOCATES VIEW OBSTETRICIANS

Not all sociologists and anthropologists are allies of midwives. Some have turned their attention to the sociology and anthropology of the natural childbirth movement. Caroline Bledsoe and Rachel Scherrer situate the rising popularity of the natural childbirth movement within safety of childbirth wrought by modern obstetrics:

> As childbearing became safer and more benign visions of nature arose, undesired outcomes of birth for women came to consist of a bad experience and psychological damage from missed bonding opportunities. Today, with safety taken for granted, the new goal has become in some sense the process itself: the experience of childbirth. . . .
>
> Birthing is depicted culturally as an individual achievement, one in which a woman should be in control of her actions.[12]

Their critical insight:

> But with *control* being such a crucial issue in cultural ideals of childbearing, the greater the expectations that a scripted birth plan creates, the greater the surety that the woman will fall short of her ideal. . . . This relegates obstetricians, who have the power to disrupt a naturalism but also to save lives if something goes wrong, to being the inevitable targets of opposition.

Specifically:

> If nature is defined as whatever obstetricians do not do, then the degree to which a birth can be called natural is inversely proportional to the degree to which an obstetrician appears to play a role. The answer to why obstetricians are described with such antipathy thus lies not in the substance of what obstetricians do that is

unnatural . . . but in the fact that obstetricians represent a woman's loss of control over the birth event.

Not surprisingly, obstetricians feel that such views represent a catch-22. Their mere presence, even when lifesaving, is not viewed positively by women swayed by the natural childbirth movement, but rather with disappointment. This is the inevitable result of a midwifery philosophy that starts with the premise that childbirth is inherently safe and has an "essence" that is violated by interventions, and that privileges process over outcome.

HOW NATURAL CHILDBIRTH BECAME A BUSINESS

Natural childbirth did not start as an industry. As explained in chapter 1, it started in the 1930s and 1940s in England as a way to encourage more births among women of the "better" classes and in the Soviet Union in response to a shortage of anesthetics. The philosophy of natural childbirth crossed the Atlantic in the 1950s and, as with many imports, was adapted to the particular needs of American women.

As noted by Paula McDonald in *Lamaze: An International History*:

> In the changed atmosphere of the late 1960s and early 1970s, the Lamaze method appeared to some childbearing women and birth activists staid and regimented, better suited to the conventional hospital setting in which it had emerged. . . . The Tennessee commune The Farm offers a particularly vivid and prominent example. The community's co-founder and midwife Ina May Gaskin strove to promote a way of birth inspired

by the counterculture. . . . Unlike the quiet, composed demeanor of Lamaze, Gaskin emphasized a sensuous, primal engagement with the act of labor, supported by what she called "spiritual midwifery." Women on The Farm and like-minded birth activists elsewhere embraced birth as an embodied experience in a way antithetical to the teachings of Lamaze and his American followers, for whom the mind's conquest of the body defined success.[13]

Childbirth in the United States in the 1950s and 1960s was, like most of contemporary medicine, afflicted with patriarchal practices that made things easier for doctors but were not beneficial, and possibly were even harmful, to women. These included putting women under general anesthesia for labor and childbirth and banning fathers from the delivery room. Natural childbirth advocates questioned those practices and eventually pushed for their end. The contemporary patient experience is far better because of them.

Natural childbirth advocates could have declared victory in the 1980s and gone home; all their demands had been met. The moment that natural childbirth became an industry was the moment that they refused to declare victory and instead moved the goalposts.

The original goalposts of the American natural childbirth movement were conscious deliveries, fathers in the delivery room, childbirth education, and research into and abolition of practices like perineal shaving and enemas that either had no benefit or were harmful. All of these happened. So the new goalposts became rejection of pain relief in childbirth, elimination of C-sections, the promotion of midwifery, doulas, and childbirth educators, and the defiance of standard obstetric and public health recommendations. In other words, the promotion of the industry and its continued existence. None of these measures had been recommended by Dick-Read or Lamaze.

This change is explained in the Lamaze *Journal of Perinatal Education*:

> Although there was a period when Lamaze . . . was accused of having sold out (the "Lamaze method" was charged by some with being a male invention meant to replace another male invention of obstetric anesthesia), in the early 1990s, the organization reinvented itself as the champion of normal birth.[14]

MIDWIVES AS THE GUARDIANS OF NORMAL BIRTH

Midwives insist they are the "guardians of normal birth."[15] I'm not sure why they're boasting, because it's actually an unwitting indictment of the problematic ethics at the heart of contemporary midwifery theory. It is fundamentally unethical for any health provider to pose as a "guardian" of a procedure.

It would be wrong for a surgeon to pose as a guardian of appendectomy; it would call into question his ability to successfully and ethically treat abdominal pain when he had a clear bias toward removing appendices. It wouldn't matter if the surgeon claimed to believe that appendectomy was the appropriate treatment for abdominal pain. We would suspect that the surgeon has his own self-interest (the surgical fee, the opportunity to hone skills, the enjoyment of performing surgery) at heart.

Similarly, if a dermatologist claimed that she was a guardian of Botox, it would call into question her ability to recommend appropriate treatment for her patients. It wouldn't matter if the dermatologist claimed to believe that every patient could benefit from an injection of Botox. We would suspect that the dermatologist had her own self-interest (her fee, gifts from drug companies, the opportunity to serve as a paid consultant) at heart.

When a midwife claims to be a guardian of normal birth, it calls into question her ability to successfully and ethically care for all pregnant women. It doesn't matter if the midwife claims to believe that normal birth is beneficial for nearly every woman. We would suspect that she had her own self-interest (her fee, professional autonomy, the enjoyment of assisting an unmedicated vaginal delivery) at heart.

Obstetricians, in contrast, are the guardians of the health and lives of mothers and babies. Their commitment is to the patients they treat, not to a particular method of treatment. Their commitment is to delivering healthy babies to healthy mothers, regardless of what it takes to make that happen. Their commitment is to people, not process.

Over the past few decades, we have come to understand the pernicious influence that outside forces can exert on health-care providers. Even something as simple and trivial as small gifts to doctors from pharmaceutical companies can affect a doctor's choice of therapy (which is why pharmaceutical companies engage in the practice in the first place). But ideology is a far more powerful source of influence than pens and calendars. It too can sway a provider's judgment to use decision-making criteria other than the best interest of the patient. That's why ideology has no place in medical care.

The central questions in caring for pregnant women should be: How can I help each individual women to remain healthy during pregnancy and childbirth, and what can I do to ensure the health of her baby? In contrast, midwives, as guardians of normal birth, view the central question as: What can I do to make this woman's birth conform to my ideal of unmedicated vaginal delivery?

Unsurprisingly, the different approaches lead to different responses in the event of complications. Since the obstetrician is committed to health, complications are acknowledged and treatments are instituted based on specific circumstances, with all options available to achieve the desired outcome.

Midwives' commitment to unmedicated vaginal birth means that complications are more likely to be ignored or denied (a "variation of normal"). Treatment options are rated by whether they are compatible with normal birth, not based on their likelihood of ensuring the health of mothers and babies.

And what about what mothers want?

That's a problem for natural childbirth advocates. As De Vries and De Vries explain in relation to childbirth educators:

> Today's women demand choice, a problematic thing for Lamaze International. Historically, we have been ambivalent about telling a woman what to do. . . . Today's rate of surgical birth points squarely to the problem with choice when it comes to having babies: Women may come to our Lamaze classes, but many of them are not choosing the Lamaze philosophy when push comes to scalpel.[16]

This elevation of process over outcome has become a deadly problem in the UK, where midwives are gatekeepers of obstetric care. A number of hospitals have experienced extraordinarily high rates of both neonatal and maternal deaths. A government-mandated investigation into deaths at the Morecambe Bay hospitals revealed:

> One interviewee told us that "there were a group of midwives who thought that normal childbirth was

the . . . be all and end all . . . at any cost . . . yeah, it does sound awful, but I think it's true—you have a normal delivery at any cost." Another interviewee ". . . was aware that there were certain midwives that would push past boundaries." A third told us that there were ". . . a couple of senior people who believed that in all sincerity they were processing the agenda as dictated at the time . . . to uphold normality."[17]

Moreover:

[M]idwives took over the risk assessment process without in many cases discussing intended care with obstetricians, and we found repeated instances of women inappropriately classified as being at low risk and managed incorrectly. [S]ome midwives would "keep other people away, 'well, we don't need to tell the doctors, we don't need to tell our colleagues, we don't need to tell anybody else that this woman is in the unit, because she's normal.'"

Midwives need to take a long, hard look at the problematic ethics of a philosophy that privileges birth process over healthy mothers and healthy babies. Rather than patting themselves on the back for being guardians of normal birth, they should be embarrassed to be caught out promoting a philosophy that places how a baby is born on an equal or greater footing with whether that baby is born healthy.

PRIVILEGING PROCESS OVER OUTCOME

It's hard to imagine anything more chilling than a midwifery paper that attempts to justify privileging process over outcome. But Marie Hastings-Tolsma and Anna G. W. Nolte, professors of midwifery, have done just that. Their piece in the journal *Midwifery* entitled "Reconceptualising Failure to Rescue in Midwifery: A Concept Analysis"[18] can be interpreted as placing the avoidance of technology *above* saving babies' lives.

The authors lay out the problem:

> Failure to rescue was developed by Silber et al. (1992) who suggested the term as an indicator of quality of care with focus on surgical patients in the inpatient setting. . . . Failure to rescue was originally conceptualised as management of complications or preventing death after a complication. . . . The original concept focused on recognition of unexpected though preventable events that influenced mortality. Subsequent effort has centred on the identification of interventions to reduce events through early recognition and the skills required to do so.

The concept of "failure to rescue" in midwifery ought to mean failure to prevent death after a complication by employing early recognition of complications and using technology to treat them. But midwives don't like technology. That leaves them open to the charge of letting babies die by refusing to use the technology that would save their lives. You or I might imagine that dead babies would cause midwives to reassess their aversion to technology. Instead it has caused them to reassess their aversion to dead babies.

How? The logical endpoint of this paper appears to be that failure to rescue women from technology is a greater calamity than failure to rescue babies from death, or even worse:

> Failure to rescue as applied to labouring women likely undermines confidence in the ability to birth spontaneously and denies women access to normal birth. Such values have been purported to be of central concern to midwives worldwide.

The authors blithely acknowledge:

> Environments with high intensity of services may have short-term value for decreasing mortality for select patients with medical complication but at what cost when applied to those who are not with risk requiring continuous monitoring?

Midwives believe that there is much more at stake than the lives of babies. They can "rescue" women from technology! They offer "the unique contribution of midwifery surveillance in prevention of failure to rescue from unnecessary interventions during childbirth."

They've squared the circle. Midwives rescue too! They just rescue women from different things. Obstetricians rescue women from horrible outcomes and midwives rescue women from interference in the birth process:

> Patients may need to be rescued from the health care system and midwives are challenged to so do. The importance of addressing maternal psychosocial and physical needs during birth is crucial, potentially pre-

venting unnecessary physical and emotional suffering where birth is perceived as traumatic.

Really? Really!

Indeed, they argue that the "process involved in midwifery care is the important phenomenon when assessing promotion of normal physiologic birth rather than the actual outcome." The authors recommend their reconceptualization:

> Failure to rescue is a crucial phenomenon in midwifery care and is central in the protection and promotion of normal birth. At a time when few experience totally physiologic birth and with evidence that interference with normal processes increases the risk for complication, midwives are challenged to consider the need to rescue women from the health care system.

I would go one step further:

Failure to rescue babies and mothers from death is an immoral, unethical phenomenon in contemporary midwifery and is central in the protection and promotion of *themselves*. Going forward, women are challenged to protect themselves from *midwives* who place their professional concerns above the lives and health of babies and mothers.

HAS MIDWIFERY MERELY REPLACED THE PATRIARCHY WITH THE MATRIARCHY?

As we've seen, the origins of the natural childbirth movement were based on deeply sexist and retrograde views of women. Although it is rarely acknowledged among contemporary natural childbirth advocates, the practice of natural childbirth is also deeply and deliberately paternalistic. Interestingly, neither Dick-Read nor Lamaze opposed the use of pain relief in labor. However, in their ideology, it was the doctor who decided, based on a woman's performance, whether she needed or deserved pain relief. At no point were laboring women asked about their own preferences or needs.

So these deeply sexist, unscientific, and patriarchal practices are at the root of natural childbirth practice. How, then, did natural childbirth come to be seen as feminist? I would argue that the primary reason is that in contemporary incarnations, women, in the form of midwives, doulas, and childbirth educators, replaced men as the people who manipulate mothers into behaving in certain ways that they have deemed acceptable. Simply put, natural childbirth has exchanged the patriarchy for the matriarchy.

That doesn't mean that contemporary female arbiters don't believe completely in their view of childbirth. Grantly Dick-Read, Lamaze, and the other male originators of natural childbirth philosophy also deeply believed that what they encouraged—a docile patient who refused pharmacological pain relief—was in the best interests of women. But natural childbirth, in its current incarnation, is still about convincing women that what's actually in the provider's best interest is in the woman's best interest.

It is in the interest of midwives, doulas, and childbirth educators to convince women not merely that they can control the pain of childbirth by preparation, but that experiencing the pain of childbirth is in itself a necessary, valuable, and healthier choice.

Most important, and most apparent in countries where midwives are gatekeepers of maternity care, like the UK and Australia, it is often the midwife who determines whether a patient needs pain relief and whether she gets it, not the patient. It is the midwife who determines whether a woman's performance in labor is successful, not the patient.

UK midwifery professor Denis Walsh is on record as condemning the British National Health Service as too quick to give in to requests for epidurals.

In a newspaper interview, Walsh said:

> A large number of women want to avoid pain, but more should be prepared to withstand it. Pain in labour is a purposeful, useful thing which has a number of benefits, such as preparing a mother for the responsibility of nurturing a newborn baby. . . .
>
> Emerging evidence shows that normal labour and birth prime the bonding areas of the mother's brain more than Caesarean or pain-free birth.[19]

The mantra of natural childbirth is choice, but the meaning of the word within the world of natural childbirth is deeply circumscribed. When midwives, doulas, and childbirth educators use the word "choice," they don't mean all possible choices that a woman might make. They mean one choice and one choice only, the choice to have a "normal" birth.

Gender scholars Annandale and Clark,[20] quoted above describing midwifery as "the largely unresearched antithesis of obstetrics," ask a critical question about contemporary midwifery: "Are midwives 'with women' or exploiting women for their own ends?"

Midwives have replaced the obstetric patriarchy with the matriarchy. In reality, midwives do exactly what they abhorred about obstetricians, insisting that they know better than the patient herself what's good for her. Natural childbirth advocates have not overthrown the "authoritative knowledge" of obstetricians, they've simply promoted themselves to the role of the authorities.

DOULAS AND CHILDBIRTH EDUCATORS

The natural childbirth industry includes not just midwives, but has grown to include doulas and childbirth educators, women who often refer to themselves as "birth workers."

Doulas and childbirth educators are not health-care providers. They typically provide no health information or care outside of pregnancy. Their purpose is to create a very specific type of birth experience, regardless of whether that experience is compatible with the health and safety of their clients. They are the childbirth equivalent of wedding planners, with one very important caveat. Unfortunately, they will plan only the wedding of *their* dreams, not the wedding of *your* dreams. If the childbirth experience of your dreams happens to coincide with the childbirth of their dreams, they'll help you.

Many birth workers go so far as to refer to themselves as "birth junkies," women obsessed with the process of birth. Even Barbara Katz Rothman, a sociologist and supporter of homebirth, has noted the unhealthy nature of this obsession. In a presentation entitled "Birth Junkies: Working Through Our Relationship to Birth,"[21] prepared for a conference of homebirth midwives, she asks: Who owns the birth experience? And she offers strategies for maintaining a nonaddictive relationship with midwifery and for responding to clients' concerns about their own birth addiction. Sadly, many doulas and childbirth educators enter relationships with patients with the primary purpose of feeding their addiction, and also validating themselves by having their own choices about childbirth mirrored back to them.

A sixteen-hour workshop is all that is required to become a certified doula or a certified childbirth educator.[22, 23] Both doulas and childbirth educators have created credentials for themselves, awarding themselves with letters after their names (CD—certified doula; CCE—certified childbirth educator). They reject outside regulation and oversight. There's not much you can do if a doula or childbirth educator offers medical information and the advice is wrong.

Doula is the Greek word for a female slave.[24] In the context of natural childbirth, a doula is a person whose sole purpose is to support the laboring mother. The increase in the number of doulas has paralleled the increase in midwives. According to DONA International, one of the leading doula certification organizations, its membership has increased from 750 in 1994 to 4,500 in 2002 to 6,154 in 2012.[25] There is a considerable body of scientific evidence suggesting that the presence of a doula can improve the childbirth experience for women, both physically and psychologically. A doula can rub a woman's back, get cool cloths for her head, and provide both companionship and empathy. The benefits exist whether the doula is a family member, friend, or hired support person.

Despite only sixteen hours of training, many doulas now represent themselves as childbirth advisers whose purpose is to facilitate unmedicated vaginal birth. In that role, the doula's primary obligation is to prevent a woman from getting adequate pain relief in labor, strongly encouraging her to manage without it. Mothers-to-be listen to doulas' advice to reject interventions ranging from prenatal testing to labor interventions designed to ensure a healthy baby to C-sections—recommendations based on nothing more than a few days of class time.

The doula's allegiance now lies with upholding the tenets of natural childbirth, not with the well-being of her patients. This is an inherent conflict of interest. Doulas have taken to the Internet, with websites, blogs, and message boards promoting unmedicated vaginal birth as an ideal to which all women should aspire (and without which, it should be noted, the doulas would have no live-lihoods).

Childbirth educators have similarly professionalized, led by Lamaze International, which derives a proportion of its income from certification fees.[26] Childbirth educators are supposed to prepare women for what to expect during childbirth, but are more likely to indoctrinate women into choosing unmedicated birth and rejecting the preventive health measures of obstetric care.

These childbirth educators, like most birth workers, subscribe to an idiosyncratic, ill-informed view of the history of obstet-rics. They characterize the last hundred years of obstetrics, which clearly shows an ever-growing body of knowledge, a greater range of tools to improve outcomes, and an extraordinary improvement in neonatal and maternal survival, as "the bad old days." The dis-tant past is constructed as a "golden age," in which our foremoth-ers in less civilized times supposedly gave birth in a physical and psychological nirvana.[27]

Both doulas and natural childbirth educators profoundly believe in the philosophy to which they subscribe. Most have already experienced an unmedicated vaginal birth themselves, and that tends to be the gateway to becoming a doula or child-birth educator. Having embraced this experience as a peak human achievement, they proselytize the value of their achievement to others—and get paid for doing so.

The Commodification of Birth

My children were born more than twenty years ago. I had four children and four birth experiences, and I think about those experiences rarely, if ever.

In my nearly thirty years of motherhood, those hours leading up to the births of my children quickly faded into insignificance compared to the reality of my children's existence: their milestones, their achievements, their personalities, their challenges, and the growth of our relationship as they changed from infants to school-age children to teenagers to adults.

I gave birth vaginally, but never even thought of considering it an achievement, since it had nothing to do with me and everything to do with luck. It is an essential part of motherhood, but I found it no more spiritual than changing diapers or driving carpool or waiting up for a child late for curfew, all equally essential to motherhood.

I don't think that my children have *ever* considered their birth experience. They neither know nor care how long my labors lasted, whether I had pain relief, if they were initially held skin to skin, or how long before they first breastfed. I'm not sure if they all know that they were breastfed.

I suspect that my experience was fairly typical for women of my generation and all preceding generations.

How did the goal of childbirth change from having a baby to having an *experience*? And how, given the purportedly sacred nature of childbirth, did it change from being an intimate experience shared only with the closest of family members and friends to a live-blogged, live-tweeted video extravaganza shared through the Internet with all 7 billion people on the planet?

It happened because the natural childbirth industry commodified birth and sold the "experience" as its primary product.

MIDWIVES, THE WEDDING PLANNERS OF BIRTH

[W]hen selecting alternative providers of birthing services, women are not simply purchasing health care, they are choosing and purchasing guides for and co-creating an event that is idealized and emotionally charged.

The above quote comes from *Great Expectations: Emotion as Central to the Experiential Consumption of Birth*[1] by Markella Rutherford and Selina Gallo-Cruz. These authors draw attention to an aspect of midwifery that we are all aware of but rarely analyze. The birth experience is a product and midwives, like any product manufacturers, are heavily engaged in marketing that product to consumers.

Rutherford and Gallo-Cruz point out the striking similarities with the marketing tactics of the wedding industry.

In conceptualizing natural birthing as an emotional and idealized consumption experience, we see that birth has come to mirror aspects of the wedding, another heavily commodified rite of passage.

Natural childbirth is not about the baby, and it isn't really about birth.

Indeed:

[T]he idealization of the birth experience offers a legitimate opportunity to orchestrate another emotional consumer experience in which the bride-now-turned-mother produces, directs, and plays the starring role.

That's what midwives are selling.

BIRTH STORIES

It is difficult to overemphasize the central role of birth stories in the promotion and marketing of natural childbirth. Many women who commit to natural childbirth do so because they envision themselves reliving the narrative of the birth stories that have inspired them, and writing their own birth story to inspire other women.

Birth stories serve multiple critical functions:

< Promotion and self-promotion
< The creation of a maternal hero ideal
< Competition with other mothers
< Confession of failure

Birth stories are to the marketing of natural childbirth as wedding magazines are to the marketing of wedding goods and services. They promote the brand; they illustrate the advantages of buying the brand; and they romanticize the benefits of the brand. They are advertisements for natural childbirth, carefully edited and curated to create a gauzy reality stripped of the mess, the pain, and the cost to the purchaser. But unlike TV commercials, they have the singular advantage of being user-generated content and therefore free.

The purveyors of wedding goods and services would give their right arms for the testimonials that the purchasers of natural childbirth goods and services offer for free. Why are natural childbirth advocates willing to promote natural childbirth? Because by doing so they are promoting themselves. Every mother is the hero of her own birth story, and birth stories follow perhaps the oldest archetype in the history of storytelling, the quest:

< The mother is "called" to have an unmedicated vaginal birth and prepares by doing "her research."
< She leaves the safety and comforts of medicated hospital birth.
< She faces tests and trials: refusal of standard preventive tests and interventions, arguments with relatives and friends about the wisdom of her choices, and the attitudes of hospital personnel, who are nearly always portrayed as unsupportive. She is tempted with offers of epidural and C-section.
< Her midwife and her doula are the sages who guide her on her quest.
< The supreme ordeal is navigating labor and "achieving" an unmedicated vaginal birth.

‹ The hero receives honor, acknowledgment, and respect for her achievement. Most important, she emerges "empowered."

If the heroic mother fantasy affected only those who sought to make themselves mothering heroes, there would be no problem. But portraying themselves as mothering heroes comes at the expense of two vulnerable groups. The first, and by far the most important, are babies. Unfortunately, they serve as little more than props in this quest story. Hence a natural childbirth advocate can be convinced to risk her child's health and sometimes even her child's life to complete her heroic quest.

The other group affected by the fantasy of the heroic mothering quest is the women who don't view mothering as a quest. They can and should ignore the women who are desperate to cast mothering as a quest and themselves as heroes, but that's harder than you might think. Why? Because some mothers, in an effort to demonstrate their own superiority, tell birth stories in an effort to shame other women who did not emulate them.

Melanie Springer Mock captures this aspect of birth stories from the perspective of an adoptive mother, a mother who does not have a birth story to tell. Her piece "Celebrating the Stories That Make Us Real"[2] reflects Mock's belief that women tell birth stories to demonstrate that they are "real" mothers, in contrast to other, presumably less authentic mothers.

[I]n many cases, they serve to undermine the value of other women's stories, of other women's experiences. I suppose that birth stories might have the power to bind women together, creating communities who have a shared experience of labor and delivering. . . . Yet too often, the competitiveness of birth narrations challenge this possibility of community. . . .

[W]hat matters most—the fact we all know, even as birth narratives suggest otherwise—is being present to our children each day after their birth. . . . Those stories about mothering—the good, the bad, the challenging, the exhilarating—are the ones we should be telling each other, for these are the stories celebrating what makes us real.

Adoptive mothers may be excused from the birth story competition because they were physically unable to give birth. But women who theoretically could have had an unmedicated vaginal birth but didn't are supposed to feel guilty. And many do.

That gives rise to an interesting subset of birth stories, the confession of failure by those who had planned to have an unmedicated birth but did not do so.

First, a very detailed description of the birth is required in order to demonstrate the multiple attempts the mother made to have the ideal birth. This includes describing the really long labor or the really long second stage, the interventions refused, and the cultural trappings employed (using a birthing pool, squatting, etc.). The purpose: to demonstrate that it was not the mother's fault that she "failed" to achieve a vaginal delivery.

Second, there are the ritual denunciations of support persons. *If only my partner, nurse, or doctor had been more supportive, this wouldn't have happened.*

Third, anything else that is now less than ideal is blamed on the failure to have a vaginal birth. Whether it's a difficult latch, not enough breast milk, or postpartum depression, it is supposedly the result of her failure to have an unmedicated vaginal delivery.

Fourth, there must be a declaration of suffering and remorse:

"I am so angry with myself," "My body failed," "I am having trouble bonding to my baby."

Finally, there must be a renewed public commitment to the ideals of natural childbirth. Generally this takes the form of pledging to have a homebirth or VBAC or both.

Here's what the mother cannot do: Be honest. She can't say, "Not everyone can have a vaginal delivery and we shouldn't be setting women up to believe that this is some sort of ideal that they should aspire to. It makes no difference whether a woman has a vaginal delivery or a C-section. It makes no difference whether a woman has a pain-racked or a painless delivery. The only thing that counts is supporting all women in doing what works for them, not insisting that every woman do what works for you."

MISTRUST

Natural childbirth originated with the publication of Grantly Dick-Read's book, *Childbirth Without Fear*, but in the intervening years, NCB advocates have made fear the centerpiece of their philosophy. Not the fear of childbirth—despite the fact that it is inherently dangerous for babies and mothers. And not the fear of pain, since only the uninformed, the weak, and the unempowered fear pain. No, the centerpiece of natural childbirth philosophy— its most potent marketing tool—is fear of doctors.

This strategy makes tremendous sense from a marketing point of view. After all, who is going to buy the services of someone who hectors you to avoid pain relief when you are in agonizing pain (a doula) unless you are afraid of something worse? And who is going to let her precious baby be delivered by someone with no medical training and quite possibly not even a high school diploma (a CPM, a homebirth midwife) unless she is convinced that the alternative is worse? Who is going to waste hundreds of dollars on "natural" pain-relieving ideas that rarely if ever work, like *Hypnobabies* audio recordings and birthing stools, unless they are told that without it, they might actually break down and ask for an epidural?

I can't think of a single prominent homebirth or natural childbirth advocate who does not work assiduously to undermine trust in obstetricians. Every homebirth and NCB book, blog, and website is predicated on the belief that obstetricians are surgeons untrained in normal birth who make millions performing unnecessary C-sections in the few moments they have each day between endless rounds of golf.

Childbirth lobbying organizations like the Childbirth Connection are front and center in the effort to destroy trust between women and obstetricians. How else to explain the endless iterations of the *Listening to Mothers* survey, a giant push-polling project that desperately seeks evidence that obstetricians are not listening to mothers and repeatedly finds that the vast majority of American mothers are very pleased with obstetric care?

Natural childbirth advocates fiercely grab on to new methods for demonizing obstetric care, such as the unproven claim that modern obstetrics causes "traumatic birth" and the hope that C-sections cause long-term health problems, which have heretofore escaped detection despite the fact that there are tens of millions of adults walking around who were born by C-section and appear to be no different from those born by vaginal delivery.

What about the spectacular advances in modern obstetrics, dropping the neonatal mortality rate by 90 percent and the maternal mortality rate by 99 percent in just a hundred years? That is simply dismissed out of hand, with claims that hospitals actually kill babies, or at least instigate the medical disasters from which obstetricians thereby appear to be "saving" babies.

Natural childbirth advocates have an "answer" for just about every objection you can name to homebirth and those answers often involve misinformation and always involve undermining women's trust in obstetricians. You need to buy books, visit websites, take classes, and pay for services, and if you don't you will be a puppet in the hands of the uncaring medical establishment.

The stakes are high. If the natural childbirth industry does not successfully create a culture of fear and suspicion, no one will pay money for their books and courses or pay hundreds of dollars for what are essentially lay companions (doulas) with no particular knowledge of childbirth and a function restricted to inculcating a fear of anyone who does have knowledge and scientific training.

When it comes to natural childbirth, follow the money. Without fear, the natural childbirth industry wouldn't profit. Therefore every woman must be convinced to approach childbirth with fear.

TRUSTING BLINDLY

What does it mean to be educated in a particular discipline? Whether that discipline is architecture, anthropology, or law, being educated generally means years of study, thousands of hours of experience, and intimate knowledge of the associated texts and research.

Medicine is like that, too. It involves four years of college, four years of medical school, three to five years of hands-on training for eighty-plus hours per week, countless textbooks, and intimate knowledge of the relevant medical literature. No layperson is educated in medicine.

When a layperson claims to be "educated" about childbirth, she certainly doesn't mean that she went to medical school, has hands-on, supervised training caring for pregnant women, or is familiar with the obstetric literature. So what does she mean?

When a layperson proudly claims to be "educated" about childbirth, she means that she has adopted a cultural construct of "education" that has little if anything to do with actual knowledge of the topic. It means that she has ignored those who have actual education and training and crowd-sourced her opinions and ideas by reading books, blogs, and websites and attending lectures and classes created by other laypeople who are often equally uninformed.

Why have natural childbirth advocates confused defiance for education?

"'Trusting Blindly Can Be the Biggest Risk of All': Organised Resistance to Childhood Vaccination in the UK"[3] explores the cultural construct of being "educated." As the title indicates, the author focuses on anti-vaccination advocacy, but the principles apply equally to natural childbirth advocacy.

When anti-vaccination or natural childbirth advocates claim to be educated, they are not talking about actual scientific knowledge. Indeed, the scientific evidence is typically ignored. The claim of being educated on vaccines or childbirth simply stands for refusal to agree with health professionals and refusal to trust them. Agreement with doctors is constructed as a negative and refusal to trust is constructed as a positive cultural attribute. As the author of the paper explains:

> Clear dichotomies are constructed between blind faith and active resistance and uncritical following and critical thinking. Non-vaccinators or those who question aspects of vaccination policy are not described in terms of class, gender, location or politics, but are "free thinkers" who have escaped from the disempowerment that is seen to characterise vaccination.

This characterization of anti-vaccination or natural childbirth advocates can be unpacked even further; not surprisingly, these advocates are portrayed as praiseworthy, and other parents denigrated.

> [I]nstead of good and bad parent categories being a function of compliance or non-compliance with vaccination advice . . . the good parent becomes one who spends the time to become informed and educated about vaccination. . . .
>
> [They] construct trust in others as passive and the easy option. Rather than trust in experts, the alternative scenario is of a parent who becomes the expert themselves, through a difficult process of personal education and empowerment.

In the world of natural childbirth, trusting experts is a mark of credulity, while ignoring expert advice is a sign of independent thinking and self-education. The woman who claims to be educated about childbirth offers as proof of this the fact that she ignores the advice of obstetricians and pediatricians and embraces the teachings of former talk-show host and B-list celebrity Ricki Lake, of laypeople like Henci Goer, or of bloggers whose only claim to expertise is that they have personally experienced childbirth a few times.

If the goal of being educated isn't acquiring knowledge, then what is it? The ultimate goal is to become "empowered":

> Finally, the moral imperative to become informed is part of a broader shift, evident in the new public health, for which some kind of empowerment, personal responsibility and participation are expressed in highly positive terms.

So natural childbirth is about the mother and how she would like to see herself, not about childbirth and not about babies. In the socially constructed world of natural childbirth advocacy, parents are divided into those (inferior) passive "sheeple" who blindly trust authority figures and (superior) rejectionists who are "educated" and "empowered" by taking "personal responsibility."

When someone tells you she is educated about childbirth, beware! In my view, there is no surer mark of lack of knowledge.

SAD ABOUT YOUR BIRTH EXPERIENCE?

What would you say if your teenage daughter confided in you that she was profoundly depressed because she did not look like a fashion model? Yes, she is thin (size 4), but not size 0, like all the actresses and models she sees in *People* magazine. Yes, she is tall (5 feet 9), but not as tall as the women she sees in *Vogue,* many of whom are over 6 feet. Yes, she is beautiful, but not as striking as the models in the magazines.

What if she told you that her inability to look like those models made her hate herself? That it's the worst thing she could possibly imagine happening to her? How about if she said that she could no longer spend time with her boyfriend because he deserved a thinner girlfriend? In fact she couldn't enjoy and didn't deserve to enjoy any aspect of her life unless and until she could look exactly like those models she so admires.

I'm going to guess that you might point out to her that being a healthy weight for her height and body type is far more important than wearing a specific clothing size. That the models that she aspires to emulate differ markedly from real women and that it makes no sense to try to emulate them. That in fact they themselves don't really look like they appear in magazines; they are airbrushed and Photoshopped to a perfection impossible to attain in real life.

I'm going to guess that you would take pains to explain to your daughter how women have been exploited by the fashion industry into feeling inferior so they will buy more clothing, more makeup, and more diet aids in a futile and psychologically harmful attempt to replicate the arbitrary standards decreed by that industry. You might even point out that this industry is profoundly antifeminist, judging women for their bodies and not their minds.

In other words, if your daughter was sad that she wasn't the ideal weight, height, and proportions decreed by the fashion industry, you would blame the industry that set her up for disappointment.

Now imagine that you are profoundly depressed that you did not have a natural childbirth. Yes, you had a healthy baby, but you did not give birth vaginally. Yes, you survived the experience, but you "gave in" and got an epidural. Sure, your baby is breastfeeding fine, but you have a lot of nipple pain, and you're sure it is because you weren't able to do the breast crawl in the operating room.

Now you view the loss of your natural birth as the worst thing that has ever happened to you. You can't enjoy your baby because you didn't really "give birth" to her; she was surgically removed like a tumor. You can no longer enjoy and don't deserve to enjoy any aspect of your life until you achieve your healing homebirth.

Imagine, in other words, that you are like this woman featured on the blog *Homebirth Cesarean*:

> *Losing the home birth was the scariest thing I could imagine.*
> *I had been preparing for this home birth the entire pregnancy.*
> *I did my prenatal yoga where I would hold incredibly uncom-*
> *fortable poses for 60 seconds, breathing through them as if they*
> *were contractions and visualizing my body opening and my*

baby being closer to me. Then squatting at the end of the session, envisioning my baby coming out and being lifted into my arms. Every single workout I did would end in happy tears because I was practicing giving birth to my baby and soon she would be on my chest.[4]

But she went past her due date, her labor stalled, and her baby's heart rate began to dip. She ended up with a C-section.

And this was my fault. My body so broken labor wouldn't start, and now it was on the verge of suffocating G. I had no choice but to give up my body for my baby. It was a moment of sacrifice: sacrifice of my dreams, of my body, of my future pregnancies and births and possibly even children.

What would I tell this mother if I had the chance?

HAVING A HEALTHY BABY IS MOST IMPORTANT

The experience you aspired to differs markedly from what real women experience, and it makes no sense, either physically or psychologically, to try to emulate those who have an idealized experience.

The women who do have the idealized experience are simply lucky—not stronger, not better made, not more deserving.

I would tell her that she has been exploited by the natural childbirth industry, an industry that sells childbirth "fashion," attempting to convince women that they need midwives, doulas, childbirth educators, hypnotherapy tapes, books, and DVDs in a futile and psychologically harmful effort to replicate an arbitrary standard decreed by an industry that makes money *only* if you accept their arbitrary standard.

And I would emphasize that the natural childbirth industry is profoundly antifeminist, judging women for the function of their bodies and not their minds. In other words,*if you are sad that you didn't have an unmedicated vaginal birth, blame the industry that set you up for disappointment, the natural childbirth industry.*

A SAFE, SANE, SATISFYING BIRTH

I offer this plan in an effort to mitigate the guilt, disappointment, and self-recrimination engendered by standard birth plans. What follows is *not* a plan to manage birth, but a plan to manage *expectations around birth* in order to ensure a safe, sane, and satisfying experience.

This is *not* a plan to achieve the birth of your dreams. The birth of your dreams exists in one and only one place—*your dreams.* Planning the birth of your dreams is the equivalent of planning to have an infant who sleeps through the night at three weeks of age. Although it could happen, it's not likely, and expecting it to happen is a virtual guarantee of frustration, disappointment, and anger.

This is *not* a plan to achieve bragging rights. In my view, birth is an intimate experience reserved for those closest to the baby and the medical professionals needed to ensure the health of the mother and baby. It is *not* an opportunity to feel superior to other women, any more than having painless periods or receiving great oral sex is a reason to feel superior to other women. It is none of their business.

This is *not* a plan to empower you. You can't be empowered by birth any more than you can be empowered by menstruation or digestion. It happens, regardless of what you think about it—or indeed, whether you think about it at all.

This *is* a plan to ensure, as much as possible, a healthy baby and a healthy, nontraumatized, happy, satisfied mother.

Here's the plan:

1. **Don't plan.** Planning your baby's birth makes as much sense as planning the weather on the day your baby is born. Because birth is a natural process, you have no control over it. You have no idea what your labor will be like, no idea what position the baby will be in, no idea how much pain you will have or how you will tolerate that pain, and no idea how or if your baby will tolerate labor. You can plan what music is on your iPod and perhaps what color Popsicles you'd like to suck on in labor. That's about it.

2. **Respect birth.** Birth is a wild, powerful, potentially life-threatening process. It's like a hurricane or a tornado. You can't control it; you just have to do what you can to stay safe and ride it out. Don't trust birth. Birth is no more trustworthy than hurricanes or tornadoes. Only a fool trusts that her thoughts can prevent a tornado from hitting her house. Sensible people go to the basement and hope that the storm passes by.

3. **Expect to experience the worst pain of your life.** There is a reason why the writers of the Bible imagined that childbirth is a punishment from God. It is widely recognized among specialists in pain management to be the worst pain you are likely ever to experience. It is absolutely essential to have realistic expectations about the pain of labor. In my experience, the single

biggest source of disappointment for women is that they believed the *lies* about pain spoon-fed to them by the natural childbirth industry: that the contractions are not pain but "surges," that there is a difference between "good" pain (childbirth) and "bad" pain (all other sources of pain), that the pain is beneficial, that birth is "orgasmic," or the racist, sexist fabrication of the originators of natural childbirth, that it is fear that leads to pain. No, the fact is, a baby's being forced from your body is the source of the pain. Do you find super-sized tampons uncomfortable? Extrapolate and you begin to get the idea.

I say this not to scare you but to prepare you. I have contempt for health-care professionals who tell you "this won't hurt" in an effort to gain your cooperation when they know it will hurt a lot. Honesty is a bedrock value in medical care. You can't trust people who lie to you about pain.

4. **Don't make any decisions about pain medication until you feel the pain.** Deciding before labor begins to refuse an epidural is the equivalent of vowing not to use an umbrella next Tuesday. You don't know what the weather will be next Tuesday, so it would be the height of foolishness to make plans before you know. The *only* people who encourage you to make decisions about pain management before you actually feel and assess the pain are people who benefit from your decision to refuse pain relief. Make decisions based on what is good for you, not what is good for them.

5. **Trust yourself.** Understand your own priorities and don't get fooled into substituting someone else's priorities for your own.

6. **Trust preventive care.** Obstetrics is, at heart, preventive care. It's all about the tests and procedures that monitor for complications so they can be managed early, long before disaster strikes. Opposing obstetric tests and procedures is like opposing colonoscopies when you are over fifty. Sure, most people who have a colonoscopy don't have colon cancer, but that doesn't mean that most colonoscopies are unnecessary. It is always better to prevent a complication then wait for it to happen.

7. **Don't keep secrets.** Obstetricians and labor nurses are not mind readers. You are a unique individual with unique experiences and fears that can impact your experience of birth. Have you been a victim of sexual assault? Do you have a fear of needles? Let your health-care providers know. Most are extremely sensitive to individual fears and will try to do what they can to mitigate those fears.

8. **Don't be confrontational.** Natural childbirth advocates encourage women to be confrontational as an effective way to undermine the trust between women and their providers. It serves the interests of natural childbirth advocates to set up barriers between you and the people who are caring for you. It does not serve your interest at all.

9. **Don't pretend that your thoughts have the power to avert or cause disaster.** Imagine if someone told you that you can cause skin cancer by wearing sunscreen and prevent it by planning not to get skin cancer. Utterly foolish, right? But that's the thinking of natural childbirth advocates who claim that thinking about complications causes complications and that

ignoring them and imagining that they won't happen will prevent them.

10. **Keep your eye on the ball.** In this case, the "ball" is a healthy mother and a healthy baby. It is not a specific birth experience. You can recover from disappointment. You will never fully recover if something goes terribly wrong.

The best way to have a safe, sane, satisfying birth is to have realistic expectations, plan on pain, decide about pain medication when you feel that pain, trust preventive care, keep your eye on the ball, and, above all, RESPECT BIRTH. It is wild, powerful, unpredictable, and unplannable, and anyone who tries to convince you otherwise is not being honest.

The Business of Breastfeeding

How did breastfeeding become a moral issue?

As a mother who breastfed four children more than two decades ago, I can tell you that this is a relatively recent development. Back when I was nursing my babies, breastfeeding was recognized as one of two excellent ways to nourish an infant. Breastfeeding was considered marginally better, but not so much so that it was worth hounding women to breastfeed. It was known to have benefits, but these paled into insignificance compared with the benefits of vaccinations or car seats or access to high-quality education.

The truth is, the moralization of breastfeeding has paralleled the monetization of breastfeeding. It wasn't until lactivism became a business that breastfeeding became a moral imperative.

MYTHS ABOUT DOCTORS AND BREASTFEEDING

Lactivists often claim that infant formula was invented even though there was no need for it, and that an unholy alliance of formula makers and physicians subsequently tricked women into believing in nonexistent benefits. But that is the exact opposite of what actually happened.

As Rima Apple explains in *Mothers and Medicine: A Social History of Infant Feeding*:

> In attempting to uncover the roots of our present circumstances, historical studies often portray women as passive in the face of medicine expertise, (male) physicians as engaged in conscious manipulation of (female) patients, or both. Although such analyses illuminate certain aspects of today's situation, they ignore many important dynamics. This is especially the case for an issue of historical and contemporary importance—infant feeding.[1]

The development of formula was not precipitated by pharmaceutical companies; rather it was precipitated by the reality that substantial numbers of women couldn't or wouldn't breastfeed their babies. Far from "creating" a need for formula, physicians, having failed to convince women that breastfeeding was a matter of life and death, were desperate to find a safe, nutritious substitute food for infants who were dying in droves.

In fact, the first true lactivists were physicians. As Jacqueline Wolf explains in the chapter "Saving Babies and Mothers: Pioneering Efforts to Decrease Infant and Maternal Mortality":

> The custom of feeding cows' milk via rags, bottles, cans and jars to babies rather than putting them to the breast became increasingly common as the last quarter of the nineteenth century progressed. . . . In 1912, disconcerted physicians complained bitterly that the breastfeeding duration rate had declined steadily since

the mid-nineteenth century. . . . A 1912 survey in
Chicago . . . [found] sixty-one percent of those women
fed their infants at least some cows' milk within weeks
of giving birth.[2]

The unwillingness of mothers to breastfeed crossed every
strata of society. This refusal to breastfeed, or at least to breastfeed exclusively, led to soaring rates of infant mortality because
unpasteurized cows' milk was contaminated.

In the early decades of the 1900s, in an effort to save infant
lives, physicians and public health officials embarked on two par-
allel campaigns, the first designed to increase rates of exclusive
breastfeeding, the second aimed at teaching women to pasteur-
ize milk. The emphasis was placed on breastfeeding, but many
women did not want to breastfeed; public health campaigns to
increase breastfeeding rates were dismal failures.

Ultimately, cows' milk was replaced by infant formula, which
more closely matches the composition of human milk, is not contaminated with harmful bacteria, and is very convenient to buy,
store, and use. The bottom line, contrary to the propaganda of the
lactivist organizations, is that breastfeeding rates did not decline
in response to the availability of breast milk substitutes. Breastfeeding rates declined substantially long before the advent of safe
substitutes.

THE HISTORY OF THE LA LECHE LEAGUE

Just as the natural childbirth industry owes its origins to religion-
inflected beliefs about the appropriate role of women, the lactation industry also owes its origins to religion-inflected beliefs
about how women should use their bodies.

In the book *La Leche League: At the Crossroads of Medicine, Feminism, and Religion,* Jule DeJager Ward explains that the La Leche League was

> founded in 1956 by a group of Catholic mothers who sought to mediate in a comprehensive way between the family and the world of modern technological medicine. . . .
>
> [A] central characteristic of La Leche League's ideology is that it was born of Catholic moral discourse on family life. . . . The League has very strong convictions about the needs of families. The League's presentations and literature carry a strong suggestion that breast feeding is obligatory. Their message is simple: Nature intended mothers to nurse their babies; therefore, mothers ought to nurse.[3]

LLL is based on Catholic theology's view of the family during this time:

> The idealization of motherhood reflects the place of Mary in Catholic popular devotion. And the approach to community strongly resembles that of the Christian Family Movement.

Indeed, the two women who recruited their friends to start the La Leche League met at a Christian Family Movement picnic, and the name of the movement was actually taken from a Catholic devotional statue of Mary, Nuestra Señora de la Leche y Buen Parto, which means Our Lady of Happy Delivery and Plentiful Milk.

So what is LLL's traditional ideology?

> The League's answer to the question "What should mothers do" is grounded in . . . the original faith community of its founders.
>
> For those women, the contents of their Catholic faith and the existential question of motherhood are interdependent.

Just as it can be read that Grantly Dick-Read created natural childbirth in opposition to women's demands for emancipation, LLL channeled the Catholic Church's opposition to women's emancipation—in particular, women's desire to work for their own economic freedom. Breastfeeding, therefore, came to be viewed as part of the Catholic mother's obligation to remain at home with her children.

Indeed, the founders of LLL were aware of the complementarity of their views and those of natural childbirth. At one of their first major meetings, in 1957, Grantly Dick-Read himself was the featured speaker.

PROFESSIONALIZING AND MONETIZING BREASTFEEDING ADVICE

LLL was and remains a volunteer organization in which women who have breastfed successfully help their friends and neighbors do the same. In 1958 they published their collective wisdom as the first edition of *The Womanly Art of Breastfeeding*[4] in loose-leaf format. Proselytizing has always been a key component of the movement.

In 1972, breastfeeding initiation rates started to rise from a nadir of less than 25 percent. The profile of the league also rose as it spread to other countries. In 1981, it was welcomed into consultative status with the United Nations Children's Fund (UNICEF).[5]

As the league gained influence, it moved to professionalize the practice of giving breastfeeding advice so that members could be paid for advice that they had previously given for free. It created the credential for the professional lactation consultant (IBCLC) and the credentialing organization.

> There are now many specially designated employment positions for IBCLCs in hospitals, clinics, nutrition programs, and in private practice. . . . The IBCLC credential identifies them as qualified to help their facilities to:
>
> < provide quality breastfeeding care;
> < develop and implement a breastfeeding protocol;
> < improve lactation knowledge and skills of other staff; and
> < become accredited under the Baby Friendly Hospital Initiative.
>
> LLLI is proud to have been a partner in this pioneering action to establish a new allied health care profession. Leaders who wish to do so now have the opportunity to move from a volunteer to a career position that allows them to continue helping mothers breastfeed their babies with the skills they have gained as LLL Leaders.[6]

The principles that characterized the organization in its earliest days—its grounding in religious belief about the role of the mother, its belief that women are obligated to breastfeed, and its zeal for proselytizing—have been transformed into a lucrative business model that makes breastfeeding promotion a source of income for many lactivists and lactivist organizations.

The desire for increased income and profits has given breast-feeding promotion a new urgency for lactivists. It's no longer merely about what is good for babies; it's also about what is good for lactivists. Unfortunately, as a result of that desire for profit, lactivists, professional and nonprofessional, have grossly inflated the benefits of breastfeeding, grossly exaggerated the "risks" of bottle-feeding, and made scare tactics and guilt the centerpiece of their efforts.

The moralization of breastfeeding parallels the monetization of breastfeeding.

Lactivists have become far more successful at promoting guilt than at promoting sustained and exclusive breastfeeding.

HOW LACTIVISTS TRY TO SCARE WOMEN

Harmony Newman explains the strategies of the lactivist movement in her dissertation "Cross-Cultural Framing Strategies of the Breastfeeding Movement and Mothers' Responses":

> Through the active construction of formula feeding as a dangerous behavior, breastfeeding activists intend to change mothers' health beliefs and behaviors such that they feel compelled to breastfeed rather than formula feed their children.[7]

Scare tactics represent the most common approach.

> Even though these arguments are portrayed as absolute, scientific fact, these arguments are better understood as a rhetorical strategy to persuade mothers of the health threats to their children. . . . In contrast to this

absolutist presentation, the evidence is more accurately described as suggestive and inconclusive.

Lactivists also invoke emotional and intellectual benefits:

This framing strategy, which constructs breastfeeding as an "act of love," puts another layer of pressure on mothers to breastfeed insofar as mothers might interpret the reverse of this argument to mean that those who fail to breastfeed their child somehow love their children less than mothers who breastfeed. Statements such as these, however, have very little evidentiary support.

These strategies are not merely scientifically inaccurate, but are also ethically fraught, because as we saw in chapter 5, they deliberately misrepresent the research. The existing scientific evidence shows that breastfeeding has real benefits, but in industrialized countries, those benefits are trivial.

Why have these scare tactics failed to increase extended breastfeeding rates? In large part it is because the scare tactics do not comport with what women have seen and experienced. Almost all women know many formula-fed babies who grew into happy, healthy, intelligent children. Indeed, many women who consider themselves happy, healthy, and intelligent were formula-fed babies. Since it is difficult to reconcile lactivists' claims with the life experience of these women, many must conclude that lactivists' claims are false or at the very least a reach.

Unfortunately, even women who know that formula-feeding is not harmful nonetheless feel incredible guilt over not breastfeeding and force themselves to attempt to breastfeed no matter the physical and emotional costs.

MONETIZING GUILT THROUGH THE BABY-FRIENDLY HOSPITAL INITIATIVE

The Baby-Friendly Hospital Initiative USA,[8] a branch of the global Baby-Friendly Hospital Initiative, is an attempt to foist guidelines created for the developing world onto women of the first world. Not surprisingly, it is led by a midwife and a lactation consultant.

The global initiative was founded in 1991 by the World Health Organization and the United Nations Children's Fund (UNICEF) and it is based on the WHO/UNICEF precepts for encouraging breastfeeding in developing countries.[9] The use of formula in these countries is extremely problematic; indeed, it can be deadly. When contaminated water is used to reconstitute powdered baby formula, serious illness is often the result. In the developing world, the WHO/UNICEF guidelines can make the difference between life and death.

Are guidelines drafted for countries where poverty is endemic, water supplies are contaminated, and starvation always a possibility, applicable to the United States? No, of course not. But the lactivism community doesn't want that fact out there. American women too must be convinced into breastfeeding by any means available. And that includes misrepresenting the risks and the state of the scientific evidence, as we can see in the BFHI literature.

> More than one million infants worldwide die every year because they are not breastfed or are given other foods too early. Millions more live in poor health, contract preventable diseases, and battle malnutrition. Although the magnitude of this death and disease is far greater in the developing world, thousands of infants in the

United States suffer the ill effects of suboptimal feeding practices. A decreased risk of diarrhea, respiratory and ear infections, and allergic skin disorders are among the many benefits of breastfeeding to infants in the industrialized world.[10]

A million infants die each year? That's right. Are any of them in the United States? No. The magnitude of death and disease is far greater in the developing world? That's right. Are any term babies dying for lack of breastfeeding in the United States? No. Decreased risk of diarrhea, respiratory and ear infections, and allergic skin disorders? Maybe (but don't let American women know that some of these claims are in doubt).

The quoted paragraph above is misleading and not strictly true, but for lactivists, the ends justify the means. And one of the ends is the monetization of guilt. The Baby-Friendly Hospital Initiative is remarkably profitable for the organization that awards the credential.

Consider the fee schedule[11] for Baby-Friendly Hospital accreditation.

Baby-Friendly USA, Inc.
Fee Schedule
Effective 7/1/2014 thru 6/30/2015

For New Facilities Entering the 4-D Pathway to Baby-Friendly Designation

Phase	Hospitals	Free Standing Birth Centers & Hospitals With Fewer Than 500 Births Per Year
Discovery	$0 Fee	$0 Fee
Development	$3,600	$2,800
Dissemination	$3,900	$3,000
Designation	$4,200	$3,200

A hospital must pay $11,700 for the designation.

As the BFHI notes:

> Fees paid by hospitals and birthing centers seeking the
> Baby-Friendly designation are the primary source of
> funding support for Baby-Friendly USA, Inc.

The biggest problem with the Baby-Friendly Hospital Initiative, though, is that it is a spectacular and expensive *failure*. That's
not surprising, since there was never any scientific evidence that
it would work in first world countries anyway.

Of course women might have told them that these efforts
were bound to fail, but no one asked them, as noted in the paper
"Rethinking Research in Breast Feeding":

> It is notable that in a field in which the behaviour and
> views of women, their families and society are so cru-
> cial, few studies incorporated an assessment of partici-
> pants' views.[12]

Lactivists only care what lactivists think.

Lactivists proclaim that women stop exclusive breastfeeding
because of lack of education, because hospitals give out formula,
because of lack of professional support, because of lack of peer support, and a myriad of other reasons. All this reflects the profound
unwillingness of breastfeeding advocates to avoid addressing the
real reasons that women stop breastfeeding or fail to start in the
first place. The truth about breastfeeding, a truth that lactivists
refuse to acknowledge, is that starting is hard, painful, frustrating, and not always logistically possible. And continuing breastfeeding is hard, sometimes painful, and incredibly inconvenient,
especially for women who work, which today is most women.

"Baby-friendly" hospital initiatives are in fact misnamed. It would be more appropriate to call them "lactivist-friendly," since the only thing they reliably do is make lactivists feel good about themselves and their own choices. No program can be "baby-friendly" if there is no evidence that it works, if it does not address the real issues, and if it shames and denigrates the mothers of those babies.

IS THE BABY-FRIENDLY HOSPITAL INITIATIVE REALLY ANYTHING BUT?

There is a real possibility that the Baby-Friendly Hospital Initiative (BFHI) may actually be harming babies.

There is not, and there can never be, anything "baby friendly" about destroying the confidence of new mothers and making them feel guilty about a decision with trivial consequences. A new paper raises the possibility that it isn't only maternal confidence that is being killed. The paper is "Deaths and Near Deaths of Healthy Newborn Infants While Bed Sharing on Maternity Wards,"[13] published in the *Journal of Perinatology*.

It starts with the obvious. Bed sharing (co-sleeping) is known to be very dangerous to babies, and the risk is highest when mothers are impaired:

> Although bed sharing with infants is well known to be hazardous, deaths and near deaths of newborn infants while bed sharing in hospitals in the United States have received little attention. . . . We report 15 deaths and 3 near deaths of healthy infants occurring during skin-to-skin contact or while bed sharing on maternity wards in the United States. Our findings suggest that

such incidents are underreported in the United States and are preventable.

What factors contributed to these fifteen deaths and two near deaths?

> In eight cases, the mother fell asleep while breastfeeding. In four cases, the mother woke up from sleep but believed her infant to be sleeping when an attendant found the infant lifeless. One or more risk factors that are known or suspected . . . were present in all cases. These included . . . maternal sedating drugs in 7 cases; cases of excessive maternal fatigue, either stated or assumed if the event occurred within 24 h of birth in 12 cases; pillows and/or other soft bedding present in 9 cases; obesity in 2 cases; maternal smoking in 2 cases; and infant swaddled in 4 cases.

In other words, mothers were encouraged to keep babies in bed with them even though multiple modifiable risk factors for infant suffocation were present, including maternal impairment due to sedating drugs or exhaustion and soft bedding. Why? To encourage breastfeeding, of course.

The author notes:

> A stated aim of BF USA [US branch of the BFHI] is to "help mothers initiate breastfeeding within one hour of birth" . . . BF USA advises that infants and mothers share a room continuously and that infants be breast fed on demand without restricting the duration of the feeding and with a minimum of 10–12 feedings in 24 hours.

As a result, hospitals have felt free to abolish well-baby nurseries, thereby reducing costs. An unholy alliance of lactivists and hospital administrators have conspired to force new mothers to keep babies with them at all times *despite* the fact that we know that such behavior is not safe for babies.

How can we prevent these entirely preventable infant deaths?

> When a mother is in close contact with her infant, one-on-one supervision of infant and mother should be undertaken by a person trained to monitor the infant's wellbeing as well as the mother's wakefulness. In many cases, nurses will be unavailable for these duties. . . . In some cases, dedicated relatives or friends might perform this function. An alternative approach would be to electronically monitor infants (heart rate or arterial saturation) with alarms referred to the nursing station to avoid disturbing parents with false alarms. This would offer considerable protection for infants in close physical contact with mothers.

Or here's a radical thought: we could mandate well-baby nurseries in all postpartum wards and allow mothers to send their babies to the nursery when they want to sleep.

It is long past time to reassess the Baby-Friendly Hospital Initiative. Anything that leads to preventable infant deaths *can't* be baby friendly.

THE COMMODIFICATION OF BREAST MILK

The commercialization of breast milk is the inevitable result of the natural parenting industry's relentless commercialization and promotion of products and services primarily to enrich itself. It's yet another example of how "natural parenting" costs a fortune, and the benefits accrue most to the members of the industry.

The philosophy that sails under the flag of "natural parenting" ought to be free, right? It was certainly free in nature. But instead it is remarkably expensive and therefore an indubitable sign of middle- and upper-class privilege.

Consider:

If breastfeeding is natural, why do we need lactation consultants? In nature, friends and family members assisted new mothers for free. Prior to the 1980s a volunteer from La Leche League would assist any woman in breastfeeding. But then La Leche League realized the money to be made by professionalizing breastfeeding advice and created the lactation consultant credential. It started an organization to administer (and charge for) the credential, and women suddenly had to pay for help they previously got for free.

It was only a matter of time before a black market in breast milk arose, so that women who couldn't make breastfeeding work by buying the services of lactation consultants could pay to buy breast milk itself. The black market in breast milk is unregulated; the milk is not screened or pasteurized, and it is nearly impossible to know if you are getting the substance you paid for.

The problems with a black market in breast milk are legion. Studies have shown that the milk is often contaminated with bacteria, including those that cause harmful illnesses.[14] Black-market breast milk is often mixed with formula or cow's milk in order to increase profits. Why would a mother feed her baby someone else's breast milk that might be filled with bacteria or corrupted with cow's milk, the very substance that these mothers were specifically trying to avoid?

Because they've been indoctrinated to believe that breast milk (even someone else's breast milk) is "liquid gold" when it is nothing of the kind. To my knowledge, there has not been even a single study showing that there is any benefit to feeding someone else's breast milk to a baby.

But that doesn't matter because parents have also been indoctrinated to believe that raising a *superior* child "naturally" is a project to be managed with lots of money. The commercialization of breast milk is merely the latest form of conspicuous consumption, easily available to the privileged and utterly out of reach of those lower on the economic scale.

In fact the only thing surprising about black-market breast milk is that it took so long for the natural parenting conspicuous consumption brigade to think of it.

PART III

A SEXIST PHILOSOPHY OF PRIVILEGE

< 10 >

How Natural Parenting Is Anti-feminist

I've been blogging about natural parenting for nearly ten years, and people often ask me if I've run out of things to write about. I never do, because natural parenting is about more than the science of parenting or the industry that promotes natural parenting. The reason parenting issues are so compelling and generate such heated emotions is that they are really about what we believe to be the proper role of women.

In my judgment, natural parenting is at its heart about relegating women to the home.

For most of human existence, women were reduced to and judged by the functions of three body parts: vagina, uterus, and breasts. Arguably the greatest civil rights achievement of the twentieth century was the emancipation of women. For all of human existence, women had been relegated to secondary, nearly subservient status. For the first time ever, some women in some societies were able to take their place alongside men, finally achieving political, intellectual, and legal equality.

Profound social change does not occur without opposition or fear. In my view, the backlash against women's emancipation has been expressed on the political right as a rise of religious fundamentalism and on the political left as the rise of natural parenting. Both function, explicitly or implicitly, to keep women in the home.

That's why it is so critical to explore these issues. Certainly it is important to ease women's minds by explaining how natural parenting subverts the existing scientific evidence. And it is also important to point out that natural parenting is a business, since we are more skeptical of claims made by businesses than by people who simply want to help. But most important of all is to understand that natural parenting has precious little to do with children and everything to do with mothers.

THE ORIGINAL PURPOSE OF NATURAL PARENTING

As we have seen, Grantly Dick-Read was painfully honest that he created the philosophy of natural childbirth as a way to keep women at home. La Leche League channeled the Catholic Church's opposition to women's desire to work while their children were small. Bill and Martha Sears describe attachment parenting as God's plan for raising children in a family where the husband is the head and the wife is subservient.

Although natural parenting is often presented as feminist (particularly natural childbirth and lactivism), the truth is it's deeply sexist and retrograde. It judges women by the function of their reproductive organs, reduces them to their biology and mandates that they fulfill the biological imperative to reproduce, ignores women's physical pain and mental health, and fetishizes the physical proximity of mother and child, thereby making work outside the home infeasible.

It is not a coincidence that natural parenting requires tremendous sacrifice on the part of the mother, and only the mother. Indeed, every element of natural parenting, extending to the rejection of vaccinations and the insistence on organic food, makes more work for mothers. Moreover, it is hardly a coincidence that the home is at the heart of natural parenting. From homebirth to homeschooling, the natural mother never has to leave the house and certainly should never be employed outside the house when her children are small.

That's not to say that every woman who embraces the tenets of natural parenting is committed to perpetuating a patriarchal society, the type of society embraced by the founders of natural childbirth, lactivism, and attachment parenting. Individual women make individual choices based on the needs of their families and their own desires. A woman can be a natural parenting advocate and a feminist, but it is important to understand that natural parenting was created and is often promoted in direct opposition to feminism.

RENDERING WOMEN'S NEEDS INVISIBLE

In natural parenting, women's needs are rendered invisible. The natural childbirth industry and its approach to the issue of pain in labor is perhaps the most obvious example of the way in which natural parenting uses several strategies to erase women's needs. To understand how these strategies work it makes sense to start with the empirical facts that most of us agree upon:

1. Childbirth is excruciatingly painful. Indeed, the pain of childbirth is so impressive that ancient cultures imagined that the only possible explanation was divine punishment of women for their transgressions.
2. Severe pain is always treated. No medical professional or pain sufferer would ever suggest that cancer pain be ignored or pain from a broken bone should go untreated.
3. Medical professionals have an obligation to treat pain. Every human being is entitled to the medical treatment of pain if that's what he or she desires.

The first strategy for rendering women's needs invisible is to insist that a mother's need for pain relief is insignificant when compared to the "risks" of epidurals. This strategy is all the more remarkable when one considers that the "risks" of epidurals are not empirical, but purely speculative. Presumably, in the natural childbirth realm, the baby has a need and a right to avoid any potentially harmful effects from epidurals that might be discovered at some unspecified future time. And that need (even though theoretical and in no way proven) trumps the mother's need for pain relief, despite the fact that pain of this magnitude would always be treated if it were from any other source.

Even when natural childbirth advocates concede that women might feel a need for pain relief, they employ a variety of strategies to diminish the importance of that need. These strategies involve:

< Blaming the woman for her own pain. If she did it "right," childbirth would not be painful.
< Blaming the woman for not using "natural" methods of pain relief, regardless of their questionable value in providing adequate relief.

< Blaming the woman for not embracing the pain as an "empowering" aspect of her biological destiny.

It makes no difference how small the risk to the baby might be, and it makes no difference how large the mother's need for pain relief might be.

The same thing is true for lactivism. To hear lactivists tell it, the benefits of breastfeeding are so large that every woman should make every possible sacrifice to breastfeed. She should ignore her own pain. She should ignore her lack of sleep and not let anyone else feed the baby. She should ignore her need to have time to herself. She should ignore the inconvenience of pumping when she returns to work. If there are difficulties with breastfeeding, she should just breastfeed "harder."

The benefits of breastfeeding wouldn't trump women's needs even if the benefits were large, but that is especially true when the benefits in first world countries are, as we have seen, very small. It is telling that no matter how minimal the benefits of breastfeeding are, lactivists assume that the baby has a greater right to small benefits than the mother has to anything else.

The willingness to render women's needs invisible obviously extends to attachment parenting. As any mother could tell you, continuous, uninterrupted proximity to infants and small children is extremely draining. No matter—in the cosmology of attachment parenting, the infant's purported need for physical closeness always trumps the mother's need for physical space and the opportunity to recover her equanimity and maintain her mental health. Similarly, a child's purported need to sleep in the parental bed is assumed to be more important than the mother's need for privacy or intimacy with her partner.

The reality is that every choice has benefits and burdens, and those benefits and burdens must be weighed against one another to best meet the needs of a woman and her children. When women's needs are rendered invisible, natural parenting advocates can act as if there is *no* benefit and only risk to employing pain relief in labor or bottle-feeding or allowing someone else to care for one's children temporarily. That's wrong and it's anti-feminist.

GLORIFYING WOMEN'S PAIN

In 2014, the website *Feminist Current* featured a powerful, thought-provoking piece entitled "Eve's Punishment Rebooted: The Ideology of Natural Birth"[1] by philosophy graduate student C. K. Egbert.

She wrote:

> There's something pornographic about the way we depict childbirth. A woman's agony becomes either the brunt of a joke, or else it is discussed as an awesome spiritual experience. . . . [W]e talk about the pain of childbirth—with few exceptions, the most excruciating, exhausting, and dangerous ordeal within human experience—as valuable in and of itself. . . .
>
> The euphemistically termed "natural childbirth" is often justified on the basis that it is a woman's choice, that pregnancy and birth is a "natural process," and that it is best for the woman and baby (both for medical reasons, and because a woman won't feel attached to her child otherwise). Put into context, these arguments ultimately boil down to "women's suffering is good."

Egbert is brutally honest about the philosophy of natural childbirth. Responding to the claim that natural childbirth is "better," she notes:

What about the argument for women's health? We probably wouldn't give much credit to an argument that we should strap patients to the operating table and refuse them anesthetic during surgery, even though general anesthetic is usually the most dangerous part of surgery. . . . Natural birth advocates are not concerned with women's welfare, because they are not advocating for safer and more effective forms of pain management; they argue they should be eliminated, because women's suffering is itself a good.

Not surprisingly, there was tremendous pushback from natural childbirth advocates to her claims, but Egbert skillfully defended her thesis when this piece was posted online.

But this isn't about the best way to give birth. It's about what significance we give to women's suffering and pain, and how that relates to women's subordination in general.

Egbert makes an interesting point, that the issue is less about giving birth and more about subordination. I doubt that many natural childbirth advocates out there would say that they believe in the subordination of women, but their practices certainly smack of this. From a distance, what separates their approach from elements of sadism? Natural childbirth promoters derive satisfaction from observing pain, suffering, or even the humiliation of other women and actively prevent them from seeking relief for their pain. Am I the only one who finds something deeply disturbing about this?

The midwives and doulas who chivvy women into refusing pain relief, who delay calling the anesthesiologist when a woman requests an epidural, who promote inadequate forms of pain relief (waterbirth, birthing balls) and praise women as "warriors" for enduring labor without pain relief are simply promoting their own beliefs and agendas. They believe that women (but not men) are improved by agonizing pain and diminished by relief. That is cruelty. And that is sexist.

IGNORING SCIENCE

When we were children, my generation was told that science and math were "too hard" for women; girls were steered away from physics and engineering toward professions like teaching and nursing. Women like me owe a deep debt to feminist pioneers who, often at great personal cost, paved the way for acceptance of women into every subject of study and every possible career.

That's why it's especially discouraging to me to find that while women are free to learn science and math, many still avoid it as "too hard." Because many women today lack a strong foundation in science and math, it is perhaps inevitable that they are drawn to pseudoscience. What's truly amazing, though, is that dismissing science has become for some a feminist statement.

I suspect that this comes from a fundamental misunderstanding about feminism. True, feminism is about choice; women can make whatever choices they deem best for themselves, regardless of society's view of what is "proper" for women. But that doesn't mean that every choice made by a woman is a feminist choice. It is not a feminist choice to wear a burka; it is not a feminist choice to remove your daughter's clitoris with a dirty razor blade; and it is not a feminist choice to declare that you are subservient to your husband.

Similarly, it is not a feminist choice to ignore science.

You have to give the feminist anti-rationalists credit for making lemonade out of lemons, though. Rather than confess to an ignorance of science, the feminist anti-rationalists declare that science is male and that women have "different ways of knowing" (i.e., intuition). That's a pretty neat trick: cloaking the sexist belief that science and math are too difficult for women under the intellectual cover of feminine intuition.

Although women have a right to have an unmedicated vaginal birth, an unmedicated vaginal birth is not a feminist statement. It is also absurd to suggest, in this age when more than half of obstetricians are female, that obstetrics is patriarchal. And now that young women are finally allowed and are being encouraged to study as much science and math as they wish, it is downright bizarre to insist that science and math aren't necessary to understand the function of the human body.

Natural childbirth is not a feminist statement, but not merely for the obvious reason that every choice made by a woman is not inherently a feminist choice. It is also not a feminist statement because natural childbirth advocacy is based primarily on misrepresenting science, statistics, and basic medical facts. Ignoring science is never a feminist choice.

POLICING WOMEN'S BODIES

It is a sad fact of history that men have spent a tremendous amount of time policing women's bodies. And an even sadder fact is that women have often been the prime enforcers in this effort.

Consider female genital mutilation. It is a practice designed by men, for men, to preserve men's sexual privileges, but it is performed exclusively by older women on female children in order to make their bodies "respectable" for men.

You might think that the time of women as enforcers of policing other women's bodies has passed. You'd be wrong. There are now entire movements devoted to policing women's bodies: natural childbirth, lactivism, and attachment parenting.

In fact, with the exception of female genital mutilation itself, it is difficult to think of historical movements that place more emphasis on the insistence that women use their bodies in the "proper" way. These philosophies are the new age iteration of age-old sexism. They function in large part to keep women trapped in the home, entirely focused on child-rearing, and incapable of pursuing the same goals as men.

I recently had something of an epiphany. I've been maintaining a blog (*The Skeptical OB*) for nearly ten years. During that time, there have been literally hundreds of thousands of comments from women all over the world. The epiphany is that most of them have been in response to or in defense of what women should or should not be doing with their bodies. Should women experience pain in labor? Do they have a right to abolish that pain? Should women breastfeed? Should women persevere if they have pain or difficulty in breastfeeding? Should women feel free to supplement or replace breastfeeding with formula? Should women carry their infants around all day? Should women have their children sleep in their bed each and every night?

My blog is noted for its full-throated condemnation of the myths and lies of the natural childbirth and lactivism movements, but in recent years I've decided I'd like it to be noted for something else: the firm conviction that natural childbirth, lactivism, and attachment parenting are anti-feminist. All three locate the center of women's worth in her body (specifically her vagina and breasts) and generate elaborate prescriptions for women's use of their own bodies that essentially control how they use their bodies every minute of every day. I firmly believe that women's bodies should be controlled by women themselves, not by groups who prescribe the "correct" way to give birth, the "correct" way to nourish a baby, and the "correct" way to nurture a baby.

In my writing, I've joked about the "sanctimommy" who has advice for everyone on every aspect of mothering. I've pointed out that a great deal of the appeal of being a part of the natural childbirth, lactivism, and attachment parenting movements is the opportunity to feel superior to other mothers and to belong to a like-minded community whose primary purpose seems to be praising themselves. Yet that is merely the incentive to joining these movements, not the purpose of them. The true purpose, sometimes conscious and sometimes unconscious, is to generate so many proscriptions around mothering that women are so busy adhering to them that they have little time left to participate in the larger world—and of course feel guilty when they do.

The leading female enforcer of policing pregnant women's bodies is homebirth guru Ina May Gaskin. She's the woman who lived most of her life in the shadow of a man who was not merely her husband, but the leader of the group to which she belongs, the Tennessee commune known as The Farm.

By her own admission, one of Gaskin's own children died at homebirth when that baby was born prematurely, on a bus, in the dead of winter on the Great Plains. Gaskin was relegated by her group to the "women's work" of midwifery, and she has done a fabulous job of making that work important and promoting it in the outside world. But no one should ever forget that Ina May Gaskin was given this job by her male-dominated group and that the only control she was allowed to have was control over other women.[2]

In an ironic twist, the current enforcers of these movements have turned to men to make the job of enforcement easier. Former New York mayor Michael Bloomberg's bizarre effort to promote breastfeeding, shaming women who want to use formula[3] by mandating that in hospitals it must be locked up, is a perfect case in point. Though the benefits of breastfeeding are small, lactivists were able to convince an elected official, in the largest and most powerful city in America, to put obstacles in the path of women who don't want to use their breasts to feed their babies.

Women have the right to control their own bodies. There's nothing feminist about policing birth, breastfeeding, or parenting.

THE VAGINAL MYSTIQUE

Betty Friedan's *The Feminine Mystique*[4] is widely credited with being one of the most influential books of the twentieth century. As *The New York Times* explains:

> That phrase, of course, became famous when "The Feminine Mystique" was published . . . to wide acclaim and huge sales, and it remains enduring shorthand for the suffocating vision of domestic goddess-hood Friedan is credited with helping demolish.[5]

But that suffocating vision of domestic goddesshood was a lot harder to kill than most of us ever imagined. In fact, it still exists, although it goes by a new name: attachment parenting.

Attachment parenting is just the feminine mystique writ large. In the 1950s, the "good" mother was obsessed with various irrelevant measures of her value, such as having the whitest wash or the cleanest floor. In the 2010s, the "good" mother is obsessed with enduring the longest labor without pain relief, never putting her child down, and never letting her children cry.

Wikipedia has an excellent synopsis of *The Feminine Mystique*, and several chapters have particular relevance to this modern-day incarnation of domestic goddesshood.

> Chapter 9: Friedan shows that advertisers tried to encourage housewives to think of themselves as professionals who needed many specialized products in order to do their jobs, while discouraging housewives from having actual careers, since that would mean they would not spend as much time and effort on housework and therefore would not buy as many household products, cutting into advertisers' profits.
>
> Chapter 10: Friedan interviews several full-time housewives, finding that although they are not fulfilled by their housework, they are all extremely busy with it. She postulates that these women unconsciously stretch their home duties to fill the time available, because the feminine mystique has taught women that this is their role, and if they ever complete their tasks they will become unneeded.[6]

The natural parenting industry, comprised of childbirth educators, doulas, midwives, lactation consultants, parenting advisors, sling manufacturers, and so forth, encourages mothers to think of themselves as needing many specialized services and products in order to be "good" mothers, while discouraging them from having actual careers, which would interfere with their ability to consume the services and goods offered by the attachment parenting industry.

Moreover, the natural parenting industry insists on practices that fill twenty-four hours in each and every day, from extended breastfeeding to constantly carrying young children to letting them sleep in the parental bed on a regular basis. Attachment parenting has insisted that this is women's role, and if women ever complete these tasks, which used to be confined to their children's infancy and toddlerhood, they will no longer be needed.

Natural parenting is obsessed with the mother's body, emphasizing the vaginal mystique, the breast mystique, and the mystique of the mother's arms. In some ways, the philosophy of attachment parenting is even more restrictive than the 1950s view of mothering. At least back then, women owned their own bodies. The 1950s emphasis was on the perfect home and lifestyle; the contemporary emphasis is on the maternal body that performs and then parents perfectly.

The philosophy of attachment parenting requires more than goods; it requires services, expensive services. The feminine mystique required purchasing the best laundry detergent and floor wax. The vaginal mystique requires a small army of service providers—childbirth educators, doulas, midwives, and lactation consultants—who charge hundreds or even thousands of dollars for their services. The products of the feminine mystique were economically within the reach of even the poorest women. The products of the vaginal mystique are so expensive that women are actually publicly soliciting on the Internet to raise money to finance things like homebirth.

Make no mistake: natural parenting and the vaginal mystique are every bit as suffocating and retrograde as the feminine mystique.

SHEILA KITZINGER, CHILDBIRTH, AND FEMINISM

Sheila Kitzinger was a brilliant and incisive cultural anthropologist and remained so until the very end.

Her last piece, an excerpt from her final book, printed in *The Daily Mail* under the title "Why Feminists HATE Natural Childbirth,"[7] is an unwitting acknowledgment of what I have been writing about for years: Natural childbirth is deeply anti-feminist.

> To my surprise, it wasn't just obstetricians who dismissed what I had to say. I also found myself in conflict with feminists, who saw birth in very simplistic terms.
>
> Why? Because they claimed it was every woman's right to give birth painlessly. . . .
>
> Polly Toynbee, writing in The Guardian, was particularly virulent, dismissing me as a lentil-eating earth goddess.
>
> "How extraordinary," she said, "that those who call themselves feminists fight for women's right to suffer and, in the process, inflict so much unnecessary suffering on women. The right to safe local anaesthetics, properly administered by experienced obstetric anaesthetists, should come first."

Kitzinger (like Ina May Gaskin) came of age when women were not valued for their intellect, talents, or character. So they made a virtue of necessity. If they were going to be judged by their biology, they would glorify their biology. Kitzinger was probably the premier biological essentialist in the natural childbirth movement. As discussed above, biological essentialism is the belief that all women have a biological essence and can find true fulfillment only through having children "as nature intended."

Kitzinger took the intellectual legacy of the profoundly sexist men who created the philosophy of natural childbirth (Grantly Dick-Read and Lamaze) and went them one better. It wasn't merely women's purpose to utilize their vaginas, uteruses, and breasts to bear and raise children, it was their glory.

Life had handed them lemons, so they made lemonade.

Kitzinger, as astute as she was, failed to recognize that natural childbirth was and remains a philosophy rooted in profound sexism. Women are no longer restricted to lemons. It is hardly surprising, then, that contemporary women no longer feel any need to pretend that lemonade tastes best or even tastes good at all.

There is no more of a need for women to glory in unmedicated childbirth than there is to glory in unmedicated painful periods. Women have replaced faux achievements with real achievements in every area of human endeavor from universities to concert halls to outer space.

Sheila Kitzinger and other early advocates of natural childbirth profoundly changed contemporary childbirth for the better by insisting that women want to remain awake, want to make their own medical decisions, and want to be accompanied by their partners. But they lost their way when they embraced the belief that women's worth is restricted to the function of their reproductive organs.

Kitzinger improved the lives of many women by taking the lemons she was given and making lemonade. She glorified childbirth in an era when women were restricted to childbirth. She never took the next step, the one that contemporary feminists took, demanding to leave the domestic sphere and take their places every field of intellectual and creative endeavor.

It is unfortunate that she failed to recognize that women are entitled to drink whatever they want, and are no longer restricted to lemonade.

THE FEMINIST CRITIQUE OF NATURAL CHILDBIRTH

When you peel back the layers of natural childbirth, lactivism, and attachment parenting, it seems that every aspect is rooted in ideas meant to keep women at home, focused primarily on children, and out of the wider world and equality with men. The philosophy of natural childbirth makes assumptions about the nature of women—how they think and how they feel, about their reaction to pain—and about the science behind childbirth itself. Feminist literature picks this apart, quite succinctly, showing how the movement is based upon assumptions about women that many do not support. Philosopher Katherine Beckett, in "Choosing Cesarean: Feminism and the Politics of Childbirth in the United States,"[8] explains:

> [Feminist] critics argue that the idealization of 'natural childbirth' rests on the assumption that both women and childbirth have a true essence or nature that is respected by the natural childbirth movement but violated by the medical establishment.

Beckett then points out that the claims of the natural childbirth industry that pain relief is pushed on women to their detriment is in direct contradiction of actual historical fact. She notes that early feminists saw pain relief, when it was first widely available in the early twentieth century, as a great political issue. If women wanted it, they should have it, they argued.

Feminist scholars criticize the reflexive rejection of pain relief, the idea that childbirth is an extreme sport or indicative of "machisma."

Beckett notes:

> In short, some feminists perceive the alternative birth movement as rigid and moralistic, insistent that giving birth 'naturally' is superior and, indeed, is a measure of a 'good mother' . . . [A]ccording to one feminist critic, the 'natural' philosophy . . . is as tyrannical and prescriptive as the medical model, but pretends not to be.

Natural childbirth consciously or unconsciously serves only to moralize the personal choices of natural parenting advocates, while denigrating the choices of most women.

THIS PHILOSOPHY HURTS WOMEN

If my email inbox is any indication, there are many women who feel like failures after giving birth by C-section. Natural childbirth advocates are quick to blame the C-section itself as a form of "birth trauma." The reality is that many women feel bad because of the incessant demonization of C-sections by the natural childbirth movement. The philosophy of natural childbirth, far from empowering women, is destructive to women's self-esteem.[9]

> Women's reports of "lower childbirth satisfaction" after cesarean should not be attributed to excessive and appropriative medical intervention. Rather, their negative evaluation of their birthing experience is produced by a cultural discourse of "natural" childbirth that encourages them to measure their labors against an inherently moralistic and ultimately pernicious ideal of birth.

The leading exponent of the critique of idealized labor is Georgetown University philosophy professor Rebecca Kukla:

For Kukla, the alternative birth movement's encouragement of such strategies as childbirth classes and birth
plans, while originally laudable in intent, is responsible for establishing "completely unrealistic expectations concerning how much control one can possibly
have over the laboring process." As a consequence, the
movement is implicated in "setting women up for feelings of failure, lack of confidence, disappointment, and
maternal inadequacy when things do not go according
to plan, even when mother and baby end up healthy."

We've already seen that Grantly Dick-Read was deeply sexist.
In this paper, I learned about the sexism of Fernand Lamaze.

According to [Sheila] Kitzinger, Lamaze consistently
ranked the women's performance in childbirth from
"excellent" to "complete failure" on the basis of their
"restlessness and screams." Those who "failed" were, he
thought, "themselves responsible because they harbored
doubts or had not practiced sufficiently," and, rather
predictably, "intellectual" women who "asked too many
questions" were considered by Lamaze to be the most
"certain to fail."

The bottom line is that natural childbirth philosophy does not
empower women. It subjugates them by "supervaluing the denigrated categories with which women have long been associated."
The philosophy of natural childbirth is just another way to accuse
women of being failures.

HOW WOMEN CAN RECLAIM THEIR AGENCY

Where did the natural childbirth and lactivism industries go so wrong?

One of the stated goals of natural childbirth and lactivism is to reclaim women's agency from doctors. Instead of doctors deciding that women should be asleep during birth, deprived of emotional support from partners, and subject to unnecessary procedures such as shaving and enemas, women insisted that it was *their right* to decide to be conscious, to be accompanied by partners, and to accept or reject procedures based on informed consent.

Instead of being convinced to forgo breastfeeding and forced to forgo it due to lack of breastfeeding support, women insisted that it was *their right* to receive encouragement and support in nourishing their infants in the way they thought best.

But both natural childbirth and lactivism went off the rails when they insisted that the only way women could reclaim their agency from doctors was to hand over that agency to midwives and lactation consultants.

Here's what childbirth and lactivism would look like if women were in charge of the decision-making:

> < All possible choices would be represented because women have a broad spectrum of needs and desires.
> < Birth plans would just as readily include maternal request C-sections as unmedicated vaginal births.
> < Pain relief would have a prominent place in birth plans, since most women find they need pain relief.
> < Women would choose how to feed their infants based on what worked for them, and they would *never* be shamed for bottle-feeding.

< Free formula would be available to those who want them.

In other words, every safe childbirth or feeding decision made by mothers would be respected by professionals and by other mothers, just in the same way that we owe respect to women for whatever decisions they make about whom or if to marry, whether or not to have children, and whether or not to work outside the home if they have children.

Decision-making would be bottom up: women would make the decisions and inform providers of their choices. Instead, in the process of women reclaiming their agency from doctors, midwives and lactation consultants swooped in to steal it from them. Within natural childbirth and lactivism, decision-making is top down. Midwives, doulas, and childbirth educators decide what a "good" or "normal" birth should look like and they impress that decision on women by claiming it is "better for baby" and "evidence based." Lactation consultants decide how babies should be fed and impress that decision on women by claiming it is "better for baby" and "evidence based."

In every case, women are deprived of agency, purportedly for their own benefit. Standards for birth or infant feeding are efforts at top-down decision-making that ignore the individual wants and needs of women and babies. Unmedicated vaginal birth is no "better for babies and mothers" than shaves or enemas. Both reflect the preferences of providers, not the needs of mothers or babies. And the Baby-Friendly Hospital Initiative is the most egregious example of depriving women of agency. Its name should be changed immediately to expunge the stench of mother-shaming, and its goals should be modified to reflect the critical role of mothers in determining what is best for them and their babies.

Women can't reclaim their agency from doctors by ceding it to midwives and lactation consultants. The guilt, self-abnegation, and torment of so many mothers reflect that fundamental reality.

NATURAL CHILDBIRTH HAS NOTHING TO DO WITH FEMINISM

Mariah Sixkiller claims she is a birth feminist.

> Birth feminists simply believe in a woman's right to make empowered choices about her birth experience. We believe a Mom should have evidence-based information about all her birth options, which all too often does not happen. We believe a Mom should be supported through her decision-making process and into the birth experience itself, which all too often does not happen. And we believe every Mom is entitled to her own choice, without judgment, whatever it may be, which all too often does not happen.[10]

But I'm an actual feminist. That's how I know that natural childbirth has nothing to do with feminism. Natural childbirth advocates don't believe in evidence; they misuse the term to promote a predetermined agenda. And they don't refrain from judging those who make anything other than preapproved, officially sanctioned choices.

Sixkiller writes about her vaginal birth after cesarean (VBAC):

> When the time came, in February 2012, I labored for four days with no medicine. I have never worked harder or experienced a more unbelievable thrill than meeting

my son that day. I felt relief, pride, strength, and elation. I felt empowered by the birth, and it changed my life for the better. My post-partum experience was amazingly positive—a sharp contrast with my first post-partum experience. And to this day, I look at my middle child with wonder and appreciation for the experience we had together—the time I gave him his life, and he gave me mine back.

I'm a feminist and what Sixkiller describes is not feminism. It's narcissism.

The technology of the twentieth century—hospital birth, epidurals, infant formula, and especially the pill—freed women from being slaves to their biology.

< I'm a feminist, and I can tell you opposition to women's emancipation is not and can never be feminist.

< I'm a feminist. That's why I spent years becoming an OB-GYN, so I could understand every aspect of childbirth and provide women with safe, satisfying births.

< I'm a feminist. That's why I object to the insistence of natural childbirth advocates to reducing birth to only the ways that a mother uses her vagina, uterus, and breasts.

< I'm a feminist. That's why I support the use of pain relief for the excruciating pain of childbirth.

< I'm a feminist. That's why I encourage women to get their medical information from medical experts, not from celebrities, cult members, and self-proclaimed experts.

< I'm a feminist. That's why I recognize that how you give birth to your child (or even if you give birth to your child) has nothing to do with your love for that child.

< I'm a proud, committed, enthusiastic feminist.

That's why I recognize that natural childbirth has nothing to do with feminism . . . and everything to do with manipulating women into accepting the profoundly misogynistic notion that women's worth is determined by their vaginas, uteruses, and breasts, instead of their intellect or the content of their character.

LOVE YOUR BODY AND YOUR BIRTH

There are countless women who hate their bodies.

Why? Because those bodies don't meet the contemporary culturally constructed ideal of female beauty.

Don't believe that the "ideal" female body is culturally constructed? Consider the Venus figures, prehistoric carved art depicting women and goddesses. As the famous Venus of Willendorf demonstrates, for most of human history, the ideal female figure looked very different from today's ideal. The prehistoric figurines have pendulous breasts, very wide hips, and large bellies.

The contemporary ideal of female beauty is dramatically different: regular features, low BMI, large breasts, thin waist. This cultural construct is everywhere you look. It's in movies and on TV, in fashion magazines, and in advertisements of products of all kinds.

The message has been received loud and clear. There is a "right" way to look and a wrong way to look. Those who don't meet the cultural construct should work assiduously, diet obsessively, exercise constantly, submit themselves to plastic surgery, squeeze themselves into "shapewear," and otherwise torture their errant bodies into the desirable ideal. And those who can't or don't submit to the ideal should hate the way they look and hate themselves for lack of willpower.

Childbirth is much the same.

The natural childbirth community has created and enforced an "ideal" birth that bears as much resemblance to childbirth in nature as Gisele Bündchen bears to the Venus of Willendorf.

The contemporary ideal of birth is an unmedicated vaginal delivery without interventions of any kind. Women don't experience pain or have contractions; they have "waves" and "surges" instead. Women don't scream, they "vocalize." They don't fear birth; fearing birth is a sign of weakness and lack of ideological fervor. They don't have complications; everything is a "variation of normal." They don't die and their babies don't die unless they are "meant to die," in which case embracing technology could not have saved them.

The message has been received loud and clear; there is a "right" way to give birth and a wrong way. Women should stoically bear excruciating pain or even pretend that the pain is orgasmic. They should risk their lives and their babies' lives to meet the ideal. Those who can't or won't submit to the ideal should hate the way they gave birth and hate themselves for lack of dedication and ideological fervor. They should embark upon another pregnancy in order to have a "healing" birth that they can brag about on blogs and message boards.

When it comes to body image, most of us finally come to understand that the culturally constructed ideal is corrosive to women's view of themselves. It leads to shame, anger, and self-loathing. Women come in all shapes and sizes. The ideal was imposed externally and serves to oppress women while simultaneously enriching the fashion, diet, and plastic surgery industries.

Hopefully, we encourage our daughters (and ourselves) to love our bodies regardless of whether they meet an externally imposed standard. We encourage or should be encouraging our daughters to subvert externally imposed standards by rejecting them. They and we should recognize that beauty comes from within and looks different on every woman.

I'd like to suggest an equally subversive response to the natural childbirth industry, an industry that promotes and profits from a culturally constructed "ideal" of childbirth. This culturally constructed ideal of unmedicated vaginal birth is corrosive to women's view of themselves. It leads to shame, anger, and self-loathing. It serves only to oppress women while simultaneously enriching midwives, doulas, childbirth educators, and purveyors of everything from natural childbirth books to plastic birthing pools.

We should be encouraging women to love their births regardless of whether they meet an externally imposed standard. We should encourage women to subvert that externally imposed standard by choosing pain relief if they have pain and want relief, technological interventions to predict and treat complications, and cesarean sections to rescue babies and mothers if necessary. We should recognize that a beautiful birth comes in a million possible iterations, from births in which no interventions are needed to those which involve every bit of technology known to mankind.

The beauty of birth resides in the arrival of a new life and the inauguration of the extraordinarily powerful mother-infant bond, which may take weeks or months to develop, but lasts a lifetime. It has nothing to do with how the baby was born; it has nothing to do with unmedicated vaginal birth; it has nothing to do with meeting a birthing "ideal" that allows women to stand on a false pedestal and look down upon her peers. You don't "rock" birth. You celebrate it—however it happens.

It's time to reject both culturally imposed standards of beauty *and* culturally imposed standards of birth.

Say no to the natural childbirth industry that wants you to feel bad about epidurals, shamed by C-sections, to loathe yourself for not having the "ideal" birth, and to redouble your efforts to have a "healing" birth next time.

Be subversive: Love your body as it is.

Be subversive: Love your birth as it is.

Women Do Not Have Other Ways of Knowing

Visit any natural childbirth blog or message board and it won't be long before you are told, "Trust your intuition, Mama!"

Why? This is yet another reason to ignore your doctor.

But why would you ignore your obstetrician, the doctor who has been highly trained in normal and abnormal childbirth, whose primary concern is to keep you healthy while delivering a healthy baby, in favor of a midwife's recommendation that differs? And why would you ignore your child's pediatrician, who tells you your baby is losing weight, whose only goal is that your child be as healthy as possible, in favor of your lactation consultant's insistence that you must breastfeed exclusively because even one bottle of formula will harm your baby?

The natural parenting industry has a two-pronged approach to addressing the conundrum of ignoring the expert in favor of the allied professional with less education, training, and skill.

The first prong is derogation of science itself; the second prong is elevation of "intuition."

*

There are many different iterations of feminism. Difference feminism is a strand that became popular in the 1980s and 1990s. It is predicated on the belief that while men and women are morally equal, they are not equivalent. While men purported value rationality and science, women value caring and intuition. According to this view, rationality is just one way to view the world, but there are "other ways of knowing" preferred by women.

The natural parenting industry has been deeply influenced by difference feminism. Rationalism, in the industry view, is the province of the patriarchy, and has unfairly become authoritative, not because it is correct, but because it is male. Women's intuition, in this view, is every bit as accurate as science.

The natural parenting industry does not reject all science. To the extent that science supports their claims, they are willing to quote scientific papers as "proof," but when it does not comport with their personal beliefs, feelings, and opinions, they reject it as inapplicable to women's bodies. Intuition, they claim, is actually a better way to predict outcomes for women and their children.

MIDWIVES AND SCIENTIFIC EVIDENCE

Midwives were initially enthusiastic about basing clinical practice on scientific evidence. That's because they had long told each other that midwifery was "science based" while obstetrics was not. As midwives Jane Munro and Helen Spiby explain in "The Nature and Use of Evidence in Midwifery Care":

> At the beginning of the evidence based practice move-
> ment, much of the midwifery profession responded
> enthusiastically to the potential for change. . . . Evidence
> based practice was seen to be offering a powerful tool to
> question and examine obstetric-led models of care that
> had dominated the previous decades.[1]

But of course modern obstetrics had always been based on scientific evidence; it was midwifery that ignored the scientific evidence in favor of ideology. Almost all practices exclusive to midwifery (as opposed to copied from obstetrics), including the veneration of unmedicated vaginal birth and waterbirth, were not evaluated scientifically before being introduced into clinical practice. No one bothered to check before making them dogma because they were based on approved ideology.

It has been quite a shock to midwives, doulas, and childbirth educators to learn that most of their own practices have never been scientifically validated. Even worse, from the point of view of ideology, their critique of modern obstetrics flies in the face of the existing scientific evidence. Therefore, as Munro and Spiby explain, "some midwives have not been so enthusiastic [about evidence based practice], viewing the drive to create and implement evidence as a threat to their clinical freedom."

As a first approach, midwives and childbirth educators have rejected the definition of evidence. As defined by David Sackett, the founder of evidence based practice, it is "the conscientious, explicit and judicious use of current best evidence in making decisions about the care of individual patients."[2] That sounds objective, and evidently objectivity is a problem. Midwives have attempted to solve that problem by insisting that evidence can be defined only in context. "Context" in this case really means "ideology."

Further reading reveals that evidence is valuable only if everyone in the group agrees, and in this case the group must include midwives, doulas, and childbirth educators, whether those opinions are based on science or not. Indeed, the scientific facts are merely one aspect of evidence. That explains the existence of otherwise inexplicable midwifery publishing, like Sara Wickham's "Evidence-Informed Midwifery":

> [T]here are as many different forms of evidence as our understanding of midwifery and women will allow us to see. . . .
>
> There is also an important distinction between the words "based" and "informed"—the latter is preferred by those who realise that midwifery is a process which is about far more than evidence.[3]

What constitutes "evidence" for Wickam? *A hodgepodge of beliefs and experiences, including intuition, a woman's personal experience, her midwife's personal experience, "body knowledge," "insight," and philosophy, among others.*

Or to put it another way, when the evidence does not support midwives' claims, they can easily wrap their ideas in muddy words such as "body knowledge" and "insight" to convince others they are "informed."

The bottom line is, many midwives, doulas, and childbirth educators use the term "scientific evidence" merely as a rhetorical device, in the same way that creationism and other forms of pseudoscience use it, while simultaneously insisting that their intuition matters more.

WHAT IS INTUITION?

In "Alternative Medicine: A Psychological Perspective," Finnish scientists Marieke Saher and Marjaana Lindeman explore the reliance on intuition in complementary and alternative medicine (CAM), which is remarkably similar to the reliance on intuition in natural parenting.

> [I]intuitive thinking is described as an unconscious, fast and effortless style of thinking, making use of such information sources as personal experiences, feelings, concrete images and narratives. Because the information processing is emotional as well as mostly unconscious, intuitive judgments are slow to change.[4]

In contrast:

> [R]ational thinking is characterised by conscious reasoning and mental effort, using all available objective information to come to a true answer, and willingness to adjust conclusions in the light of new facts.

The beauty of intuition when it comes to medical issues is that it allows laypeople to believe that they are "experts" in their own health and that they do not need doctors or other rational thinkers to advise them.

According to Saher and Lindeman:

> CAM messages [like those of natural childbirth] favour familiar concepts ("naturalness"), similarity, personal experience and testimonials over abstract concepts like general principles and probabilities.

The reliance on intuition is a central defect in contemporary midwifery theory, since intuition is notoriously inaccurate. In *Intuition: Its Powers and Perils,*[5] David G. Myers explores this issue in detail. In the chapter entitled "Intuitions about Reality," Myers examines the many reasons why intuition is often wrong. One of the main sources of error is what he terms "belief perseverance."

> "We hear and apprehend only what we already half know," commented Henry David Thoreau. Experiments suggest how right Thoreau was. In one experiment, students in favor of and opposed to capital punishment were shown findings of two research studies, one confirming and the other disconfirming their preexisting beliefs about capital punishment's supposed deterrent effect. Both groups readily accepted the evidence that confirmed their view but sharply criticized the evidence that challenged it.

Intuition is not "another way of knowing." It is just another source of potentially erroneous beliefs.

COGNITIVE ERRORS AND NATURAL CHILDBIRTH

Psychologists Marjaana Lindeman and Kia Aarnio, in their paper "Superstitious, Magical, and Paranormal Beliefs: An Integrative Model,"[6] postulate that believers in superstition, paranormal phenomena, and pseudoscience make similar cognitive errors, errors that can be characterized as a holdover of the errors of reasoning made by children still learning about the natural world.

For most adults, such errors are usually corrected by giving preference to analytical thinking. While belief in healing "energies" or healing thoughts may have appeal, such beliefs are clearly contradicted by what we know about physics and biology. But those who give priority to intuition and those who lack understanding of physics and biology are far more likely to accept belief in pseudoscience.

Believers in pseudoscience don't hide their reliance on intuition. Indeed, they are quite clear in giving preference to intuition over analytical thinking and represent intuition as an equally valid way of knowing about the world. Jenny McCarthy based her anti-vaccine advocacy on her intuition that vaccines had given her child autism. Many natural childbirth advocates rely on intuition to justify risky childbirth choices. Yet, far from being beneficial, this overt reliance on intuition leads to a plethora of false beliefs.

In *Spiritual Midwifery*, Ina May Gaskin offers this delicious bit of goofiness:

> We have found that there are laws as constant as the laws of physics, electricity, or astronomy whose influence on the process of the birthing cannot be ignored. The midwife or doctor attending births must be flexible enough to discover the way these laws work and learn how to work with them. Pregnant and birthing mothers are elemental forces, in the same sense that gravity, thunderstorms, earthquakes, and hurricanes are elemental forces. In order to understand the laws of their energy flow, you have to love and respect them for their magnificence at the same time that you study them with the accuracy of a true scientist. A midwife or obstetrician needs to understand about how the energy of childbirth flows—to not know is to be like a physicist who doesn't understand about gravity.[7]

Mysterious forces? Energy flow?

Anyone know what she is actually talking about? Me neither.

Natural childbirth advocacy is explicit in privileging intuition above analytical thinking. According to Robbie Davis-Floyd, intuition *is* authoritative knowledge. She explains that for "postmodern" midwives:

> Intuition . . . emerges out of their own inner connect-
> edness to the deepest bodily and spiritual aspects of
> their being, as well as out of their physical and psy-
> chic connections to the mother and the child. The
> trustworthiness of intuition is intrinsically related to
> its emergence from that matrix of physical, emotional,
> and spiritual connection—a matrix that gives intuition
> more power and credibility, in these midwives' eyes,
> than the information that arises from the technologies
> of separation. . . . [T]heir deep, connective, woman-
> to-woman webs, woven so lovingly in a society that
> grants those connections no authority of knowledge
> and precious little conceptual reality, hold rich poten-
> tial for restoring the balance of intimacy to the multiple
> alienations of technocratic life.[8]

The cognitive errors that constitute natural childbirth advocacy are summed up in the exhortation to "trust birth." Birth, a natural process, is portrayed as a living entity capable of inspiring, expecting, and rewarding trust. Implicit in the call to trust birth is the belief that specific thoughts can bring about specific outcomes. Ultimately, though, privileging intuition reflects a deep desire to ignore the fact that the most cherished beliefs of natural childbirth advocacy do not comport with the scientific evidence.

THE DUNNING-KRUGER EFFECT

This preference for intuition over scientific evidence is aided and abetted by a basic lack of knowledge among professional advocates of natural childbirth, lactivism, and attachment parenting. As we have seen, most of what passes for "knowledge" within these communities is factually false. This basic lack of accurate information is compounded by the tendency of people who know the least about a topic to believe they know the most. This tendency is known as the Dunning-Kruger effect.

The trouble with ignorance is that it feels so much like expertise. So says psychology professor Dr. David Dunning. He ought to know.

> In 1999, in the *Journal of Personality and Social Psychology*, my then graduate student Justin Kruger and I published a paper that documented how, in many areas of life, incompetent people do not recognize—scratch that, cannot recognize—just how incompetent they are, a phenomenon that has come to be known as the Dunning-Kruger effect. Logic itself almost demands this lack of self-insight: For poor performers to recognize their ineptitude would require them to possess the very expertise they lack. To know how skilled or unskilled you are at using the rules of grammar, for instance, you must have a good working knowledge of those rules, an impossibility among the incompetent.[9]

Or, for instance, to know how knowledgeable or ignorant you are about childbirth, you have to have a good working knowledge of modern obstetrics, including both normal and abnormal childbirth. Paradoxically:

What's curious is that, in many cases, incompetence does not leave people disoriented, perplexed, or cautious. Instead, the incompetent are often blessed with an inappropriate confidence, buoyed by something that feels to them like knowledge.

Many midwives, doulas, and childbirth educators have an inappropriate level of confidence despite their own lack of knowledge, and a significant proportion of lay advocates suffer from the delusion of believing themselves "knowledgeable" after having done "their research." The world of celebrity natural childbirth and homebirth advocates is filled with what Dunning calls "confident idiots."

How do people become confident idiots?

> Very young children . . . carry misbeliefs that they will harbor, to some degree, for the rest of their lives. Asked why trees produce oxygen, children say they do so to allow animals to breathe. . . . This purpose-driven misconception wreaks particular havoc on attempts to teach one of the most important concepts in modern science: evolutionary theory. Even laypeople who endorse the theory often believe a false version of it. They ascribe a level of agency and organization to evolution that is just not there.

Hence natural childbirth and natural parenting advocates claim that women are "perfectly evolved" for childbirth or that women who breastfeed "always" have enough breast milk.

The reality is that childbirth and breastfeeding have always been and are *still* governed by random differences and natural selection. Some pregnancies are too short, some pregnancies are too long. One out of 20 women cannot produce enough milk to nourish her baby. The idea that "the baby knows when to be born" is a paradigmatic example of the purpose-driven misbelief, similar to "breech is just a variation of normal" to "you can't grow a baby too big to birth vaginally."

Even more important:

> Some of our most stubborn misbeliefs arise . . . from the very values and philosophies that define who we are as individuals. Each of us possesses certain foundational beliefs—narratives about the self, ideas about the social order—that essentially cannot be violated: To contradict them would call into question our very self-worth.

The foundational belief of natural childbirth, lactivism, and natural parenting is "My birth, feeding and parenting choices make me a better mother than everyone else." Many natural childbirth advocates reject out of hand any evidence that threatens this foundational belief. Hence the epidemic of deleting and banning that afflicts natural childbirth websites and message boards.

How can we combat the epidemic of misbelief promoted by natural parenting advocates? Dunning advocates a general strategy that can be applied to natural childbirth advocacy:

> For individuals, the trick is to be your own devil's advocate: to think through how your favored conclusions might be misguided; to ask yourself how you might be wrong, or how things might turn out differently from what you expect. . . . And lastly: Seek advice. Other

people may have their own misbeliefs, but a discussion can often be sufficient to rid a serious person of his or her most egregious misconceptions.

Of course natural childbirth advocates have already cleverly "immunized" their followers against such a strategy. According to them, you should never ask yourself how you might be wrong because questioning birth inevitably leads to poor outcomes. "Trust birth!" sounds better than "Don't think!" but it means exactly the same thing.

< 12 >

Sanctimommies and the Joys of Shaming

How many times have you heard a lactivist, birth activist, or attachment parenting proponent who insists something like this:

Honestly, I don't understand why other mothers think that I am judging them. If they want to raise their children by doing whatever is easiest for them instead of what's best for their babies, that's their decision and I don't question it. I understand that some women love their jobs more than their children, and after all, who wouldn't if she had some fancy-pants career where she made tons of money. It probably makes more sense to her to put money ahead of her children's well-being.

Take my next-door neighbor, for example. She makes oodles of money practicing law and leaves her baby each and every day in the care of strangers. I am impressed that her baby welcomes her home by reaching out to her, smiling and giggling. Fortunately, nature designed babies to recognize their mothers, no matter how little time those mothers spend caring for their children.

I'll admit that I find it harder to understand how women who aren't even working give up on breastfeeding so easily, or refuse to allow their children to sleep in the family bed. What's so valuable about their time or convenience, anyway? But I keep my opinion to myself. I don't let on that I am perfectly aware that there is no such thing as a breastfeeding difficulty that can't be overcome with enough love and dedication. When other women claim they had a low milk supply or that breastfeeding was excruciatingly painful, I merely feel sad that they never had the unique opportunity to bond with their children that only breast-feeding offers.

And when it comes to childbirth, how can I possibly judge other women who haven't taken the time to educate themselves the way that I have? I've read Henci Goer's book three times, and Ina May Gaskin is my idol. Everyone knows that the first step to becoming educated on a topic is to join an Internet mes-sage board. If I hadn't joined the message boards at Mothering .com, I probably wouldn't have known that birth is inherently safe and that all that stuff about "risk" was made up by doctors trying to steal business from midwives.

The uneducated women who don't understand this can't be blamed for acting like birth is some sort of disease and needs to take place in a hospital. Of course they give in and get an epi-dural at the drop of a hat because they don't realize that there's a difference between good pain and bad pain. And they don't even understand the real risks of epidurals.

Oh, and don't accuse me of looking down on women who've had C-sections. Sure, they didn't actually give birth, and they have missed out on the peak experience of a woman's life, but is that their fault? I know that almost all C-sections are unneces-

sary, but those poor women actually think that the C-section "saved" their baby's life.

I don't judge them, but I do think that I have a responsibility to open their eyes to the ways in which they have been misled. It would be wrong for me to refrain from enlightening them merely because it might hurt their feelings. Women need to understand that anyone who thinks her C-section was "medically necessary" is being duped by those who seek to medicalize childbirth for their own benefit.

Many women don't realize it, but if they had more encouragement, they'd happily do what's best for their babies. That's why I tell my birth story to everyone, whether they want to hear it or not. It may seem unbelievable, but it's often the very first time they've heard that they could have been empowered like me if only they'd made the same decisions I made.

And let's face it, women don't get enough encouragement to breastfeed. Some women actually think that a baby who is fed artificial milk (formula) can be as healthy as a baby fed with breast milk as nature intended. I consider it my duty to broadcast the dangers of formula-feeding far and wide. It's unfortunate that we have to scare mothers into doing what's best by exaggerating the benefits of breastfeeding, but everyone knows that the ends justify the means.

Please do not accuse me of judging those other mothers who don't love their children as much as I love mine. I'm well aware that different ways of mothering are right for different families. Of course women who are obsessed with their own convenience find that bottle-feeding is right for them and their families. Obviously women who have been duped by doctors into fearing birth are going to find that hospital birth is right for them. And inevitably those who aren't really attached to their children are not going to be comfortable with attachment parenting.

I just want to be clear:

To those women who haven't really given birth because they've had a C-section, to those women who gave in to the pain and got an epidural, to anyone who doesn't understand that only breastfed babies are truly bonded to their mothers . . .

I am so not judging you.

SANCTIMOMMY

There's a new mother on the block, and she's cheerfully terrorizing everyone else. Meet . . . Sanctimommy!

Sanctimommy knows how you should raise your children. Specifically, she knows what foods they should eat, what toys they should be allowed to play with; heck, Sanctimommy even knows how you should have given birth.

The best part about Sanctimommy is that she is always ready to share her wisdom with the rest of us. She doesn't hesitate to point out the deficiencies of your parenting practices (in other words, how your parenting choices differ from hers). She doesn't hesitate to make dire predictions about what the future holds for your children ("You give him a pacifier? You know he's never going to be able to . . ."). She never hesitates to bemoan your lack of understanding of the key issues of child-rearing, letting you know that you are not as "informed" as she is.

My personal observation on the behavior of sanctimommies in their natural habitat of parenting blogs, Facebook pages, and message boards is that they tend to suffer from overwhelmingly ostentatious "sadness." They are so "sad" for you that you don't know enough. They are so "sad" for your children that you are not parenting the way they prescribe.

Sanctimommy has lots of all-purpose rules for parenting. No

need to tailor parenting choices to the personality and needs of the individual child. All childbirth should be unmedicated; all children should be breastfed for the prescribed amount of time; all children should be carried; every child should sleep in the family bed. There's a rule for every behavior and every situation—the same rule for every child and every family.

Despite her apparent self-assurance, Sanctimommy needs constant validation and she intends to get it from you. And your parenting choices serve as the perfect foil for Sanctimommy, since she can criticize them and you.

Sanctimommy is quick to take offense. In fact she is always sure that she is being "disrespected" by those who don't make the same choices.

Sanctimommy is sure that she is being persecuted. Mothers who don't agree with her are accused of interfering with her choices even if you have no interest in her choices at all.

Fundamentally, Sanctimommy cannot abide uncertainty, and if there ever was a job fraught with uncertainty, it is motherhood. It is difficult to get feedback on job performance from children. Children live in the moment, are overwhelmed with their own needs, and don't take the long view.

Children don't tell you whether being allowed in the parental bed promotes security or inability to manage separation. They don't tell you whether efforts to promote their self-esteem work or promote narcissism instead. They don't thank you for discipline and they don't applaud your performance. In fact, it often turns out that your best moments as a mother were the ones that your children appeared at the time to hate the most.

All mothers must cope with this uncertainty, but some are more challenged than others. Sanctimommies deal with uncertainty by pretending that it doesn't exist. They adopt all-purpose rules for parenting and insist that following them demonstrates unequivocally that they are doing the right thing (and, inevitably, if you don't agree, you are wrong).

And because they are so insecure, they cannot resist interrogating other mothers and demeaning their choices. Had an epidural? Too bad you gave in to the pain. Stopped breastfeeding before age two (or three or four)? How sad that you didn't try hard enough. Your children's food is not 100 percent organic? How unfortunate that you don't care enough about your children to go the extra mile.

Ironically, Sanctimommy's choices don't necessarily reflect what is best for her children. They don't reflect the fact that children are individual human beings with individual needs and desires. There is no one-size-fits-all parenting formula, and pretending that there is ignores the specific needs of a specific child. Sanctimommy's choices are all about her—her need for reassurance and her inability to tolerate unpredictability.

MOTHERHOOD AS PERFORMANCE ART

The new moralism that defines motherhood promotes the personal preferences of a select group of women—well-off white women from first world countries. Indeed, mothering is now measured by a set of socially sanctioned "performances" at purported critical moments. Philosophy professor Rebecca Kukla, mentioned in chapter 6, has written a fascinating article entitled "Measuring Motherhood"[1] examining the middle-class penchant of evaluating other women's mothering by "signal moments."

> As a culture, we have a tendency to measure motherhood in terms of a set of signal moments that have become the focus of special social attention and anxi-

ety; we interpret these as emblematic summations of women's mothering abilities. Women's performances during these moments can seem to exhaust the story of mothering, and mothers often internalize these measures and evaluate their own mothering in terms of them. "Good" mothers . . . give birth vaginally without pain medication, they do not offer their child an artificial nipple during the first six months, they feed their children maximally nutritious meals with every bite, and so on.

In other words, mothering has been reduced to a set of achievement tests that can be passed or failed. Among those achievement tests are birth and breastfeeding.

[W]e have elevated the symbolic importance of birth to the point where it appears to serve as a make-or-break test of a woman's mothering abilities. If she manages her birth "successfully," . . . then she proves her maternal bona fides and initiates a lifetime of proper mothering. If, on the other hand, she fails at these tasks during labor, she reveals herself as selfish or undisciplined and risks deforming her baby's character, health, and emotional well-being, while putting her bond with her child in permanent jeopardy.

Yet these claims have no basis in fact:

[R]eal risks and their sizes do not seem to be of interest to the lay critics of mothers' birth choices, who appear quite content with hand-waving references to gains and harms. . . . [I]t is hard not to conclude that the main normative standards at play are ideological, not medical. . . . What is at stake is not the health of babies but an image of proper motherhood, combined with the idea that birth should function as a symbolic spectacle of such motherhood.

Lactivists also make claims that have no basis in scientific fact:

North American breast-feeding promotional materials consistently emphasize exclusive breast-feeding, as opposed to the more productive message that the more breast milk babies receive, the better. "Does one bottle of formula make that much difference? We wish we could say that it doesn't," states La Leche League, rather disingenuously, in their breast-feeding guide, "but we can't."

The bottom line is that a small group of privileged women hold their own choices regarding birth and infant feeding up as standards to which all women should aspire. This is wrong on several levels. There is no objective evidence that the claims of "natural" childbirth advocates and lactivists are true. There is no objective evidence that single moments of motherhood determine the long-term well-being of a child or determine the strength of the mother-child bond. In fact, insisting that the cultural rituals of a privileged group of women are the standards to which all other women should aspire reinforces existing cultural and economic prejudices.

PARENTAL TRIBALISM

Imagine a cocktail party where everyone introduced him or herself with reference to a car.

> *"Hi, I'm Debbie, and I drive a Ford Explorer."*
>
> *"Nice to meet you, Debbie. I'm Karen and I drive a Lexus RX 350. Let me introduce Kathy; she drives a Subaru. And here's Margie. She drives a Ford Explorer just like you."*
>
> *"Hi, Margie. I'm so glad to meet someone else who drives a Ford Explorer. It can be tough to be a Ford driver in this culture when no one else cares enough about their country to buy American cars."*

What might we conclude from this brief exchange? First, it is clear that the people in this group have constructed their identity around car ownership, not simply differentiating between those who own cars and those who don't, but tying identity directly to specific brands. Second, even in this short exchange, we can see that identity creation through brand choice leads to a form of security, through a sense of belonging to a self-chosen group. Third, although the car appears to be central, this is not about cars at all; it is really about self-definition.

It sounds ludicrous to create an identity around car brands, doesn't it? Yet it is strikingly similar to the current penchant for creating identity around specific parenting choices, also known as parental tribalism. According to Jan Macvarish of the Centre for Parenting Culture Studies,[2] parental tribalism involves constructing an identity around parental choices, specifically: constructing an identity centered on differentiating themselves from parents who make different choices.

Strikingly, many of these choices, although they appear to

concern the well-being of children, are really about the self-image of parents. As Macvarish explains:

> [T]he focus on identities reflects adult needs for security and belonging and, although the child appears to be symbolically central, in fact the cultural politics of parents' self-definition have eclipsed a concern with the needs of children.

As with all forms of tribalism, parental tribalism leads to conflicts:

> [T]there is a frailty and sometimes hostility in real or imagined encounters between parents, where the parenting behaviour of one can either reinforce or threaten the identity of another.

Websites and publications concerned with attachment parenting, natural childbirth, and lactivism emphasize and encourage this hostility. There is an almost paranoid certainty that other mothers are watching and criticizing. The resultant defensiveness is the true source of the hostility. By aggressively promoting their own choices, demeaning the choices of other mothers, and insisting that anyone who makes different choices is implicitly criticizing them, advocates of attachment parenting, natural childbirth, lactivism, and so forth encourage the very conflicts that they claim to deplore.

These conflicts do not benefit children, anyone's children, in any way. That's not surprising, since they're not about children, but about parental self-image. Indeed, constructing identity around parenting choices has the potential to harm children by ignoring the actual needs of children in favor of promoting the mother's sense of security and belonging.

MOTHERHOOD AND THE TYRANNY OF THE N-WORDS

Words have power. The two ugliest N-words in contemporary parenting are these: "normal" and "natural."

There is a fundamental ambiguity between normal as "common" and normal as "morally preferable." When natural childbirth advocates and lactivists use the word "normal," they mean morally preferable or normative. The word "natural" is used in the same way, and it too embodies a fundamental ambiguity between natural as "the absence of technology" and natural as "a state of perfection that can only be marred by technology." The second use is embodied in the naturalistic fallacy that undergirds so much of alternative health and quackery, the belief that because something is a certain way in nature, it ought to be that way always.

When birth activists promote natural birth or normal birth, they are using the N-words as normative and morally preferable. Natural childbirth is presented as better, safer, and healthier than birth with technology. It's not merely natural, it's normal too, the way that birth is supposed to be. Anyone who deviates from natural childbirth has failed her child in a fundamental way.

When lactivists promote normalizing breastfeeding, they are also using an N-word to signify normative and morally preferable. Breastfeeding is routinely presented as best, just in case calling it natural and normal did not convey that good mothers breastfeed exclusively. Anyone who deviates from breastfeeding exclusively has failed her child in a fundamental way.

Birth and breastfeeding advocates are aware that describing

childbirth and breastfeeding in these ways is mean, creating two classes of mothers, good mothers and bad mothers. They want to use these terms viciously, but they don't want to be accused of doing so. Therefore they exploit the fundamental ambiguity to create plausible deniability. No, no, no, they don't mean that normal birth is better; they just mean that it is the common way to give birth. No, no, no, they're not trying to shame formula-feeding mothers, they're simply pointing out that breastfeeding is the normal and natural way to feed an infant.

We shouldn't let them get away with it.

When used in the context of mothering, N-words are explosive and destructive, so let's not use them. I implore people to think carefully before employing the words "normal" or "natural" to describe either childbirth or breastfeeding. We should strike the term "normalize" entirely from any discussions about mothers.

Words have power, and those who believe they are using the N-words to signify common or expected should keep that ambiguity in mind. Otherwise they are contributing to the ugly effort by some mothers to denigrate other mothers. Better to be precise and kind than inadvertently mean and shaming.

BABIES, HOSTAGES IN THE MOMMY WARS

The mommy wars are fights to the death.

No, not the deaths of the participants, but the deaths of confidence in their ability to mother their children.

Wait, what? You thought that the mommy wars were about children and their well-being. How naive! Yes, children are involved in the mommy wars, but unfortunately their role is as hostages.

The mommy wars are about one thing, and one thing only: Who is the best mother?

Given the viciousness with which the mommy wars are fought, you might think there was an actual award at stake, a Mommy Nobel Prize, complete with international recognition, adulation, and a cash annuity. The stakes are far smaller, though every bit as important to the participants. What's at stake is who can claim the designation of "best mother" within the social circle of other mothers.

Wait, what? You thought that the best mother is the one who raises healthy, happy children?

How naive! Looking at the children leaves much too much to chance.

In the first place, it is difficult to point to one baby as happier than all the others. Most babies are happy and healthy when given love. Why not wait until children are older to determine who is the best mother? Even those who are most adamant that natural childbirth, breastfeeding, and attachment parenting produce the best, most accomplished, most well-adjusted children recognize that the "best" parental inputs don't ensure the "best" outcome. It is therefore critically important to judge mothers by the process, which can be controlled, and not the outcome, which cannot.

According to natural childbirth advocates, unmedicated vaginal birth produces the healthiest, happiest, most accomplished children. But look at all the teens in a high school class. Can you tell whose mothers had epidurals or C-sections? No, you can't.

According to lactivists, breastfeeding produces the healthiest, happiest, most accomplished children. But look at an Ivy League graduating class. Can you tell whose mothers breastfed them and for how long? No, you can't.

According to advocates of intensive mothering, attachment parenting ("baby wearing," extended breastfeeding, family bed) produces the healthiest, happiest, most accomplished children. But look at winners of the Nobel Prize. Can you tell whose mothers practiced attachment parenting? No, you can't.

Given this reality, is it any wonder that combatants in the mommy wars are obsessed with process and ignore outcome?

That's not to say that children aren't involved in the mommy wars; they are, but their role is as hostages, props for their mothers to act upon, without regard for what is actually best for them.

The truth is that "Who is the best mother?" is the wrong question entirely.

Each child has only one mother and does not compare his/her mother to other mothers. The competition between mothers is irrelevant to children. What counts for them is whether *their* mother is meeting *their* needs. The secret of mothering is not comparing yourself to other mothers, but asking yourself, "Am I doing my best to provide what my child needs?"

There is no reason to ignore your own needs, either. If you have unbearable pain in labor, use pain relief; if you need medication incompatible with breastfeeding for your physical and mental health, formula-feed; if you and your partner want to keep your bed for yourself, do that. The truth is that none of these choices determines whether your children will be happy and healthy, let alone accomplished.

The sad fact is that many mommy bloggers, mommy message boards, and medical paraprofessionals are *mommy warmongers*. They encourage the vicious efforts of some women to destroy the mothering confidence of other women because it benefits them. Perhaps they are mothers themselves and can bolster their self-esteem only by battering the self-esteem of others. Perhaps they fuel their blog (and in some cases their blog income) by promoting an us-against-them mentality that makes participants feel good but does nothing for children. Perhaps their entire business model (doulas, lactation consultants, etc.) depends on convincing women that buying their services will ensure mothering superiority.

It is widely recognized that we have been raising a generation of children many of whom are entitled, unable to tolerate disappointment or failure, and incapable of separating from their parents and shouldering adult responsibilities on their own. Could that be due in part to the fact that we have been raising children as hostages in the mommy wars, acted *upon* by mothers determined to demonstrate their mothering superiority, rather than raised with their own needs in mind? It's too soon to say, but it is certainly worth considering.

If we cared about children, as we claim that we do, we would be spending a lot more time individualizing mothering and a lot less time creating one-size-fits-all prescriptions (natural childbirth, breastfeeding, attachment parenting) for being the "best" mother. We would be spending a lot more time supporting women in the choices that are best for *their* children, not denigrating them for failing to mirror the choices we believe to be best for *our* children.

It is my belief that the best mother is the one who cares deeply for her child and lets her child know it. It isn't natural childbirth or breastfeeding or attachment parenting that makes a good mother . . .

It is love.

NATURAL CHILDBIRTH, A PHILOSOPHY OF PRIVILEGE

Natural does not have much resonance among women of other cultures, nor among women of color within first world countries. The preference for "natural" is about and absolutely depends upon social privilege.

Political scientist Candace Johnson[3] explores the role of "nat-

ural" childbirth as a philosophy of privilege in contemporary society. She starts by framing the question:

> [W]hy do some women (mostly privileged and in
> developed countries) demand less medical interven-
> tion in pregnancy and childbirth, while others (mostly
> vulnerable women in both developed and developing
> countries) demand more? Why do the former, privi-
> leged women, tend to express their resistance to medi-
> cal intervention in the language of "nature," "tradition,"
> and "normalcy"?

The answer?

> The evidence seems to suggest that arguments about the
> negative impact of medical intervention in the lives of
> women, "medicalization," seem to resonate only among
> privileged populations. . . .
>
> In poor countries, communities or under-serviced
> areas, medical care is a necessity, upon which exercise
> of agency and autonomy is contingent. But the refusal
> of pharmaceuticals and clinical care among affluent or
> well-accommodated (by a universal health system, for
> example) women is at once a form of political resistance
> and an assertion of identity.

It is precisely this reason—that rejection of medicalization is
an assertion of identity—that explains its restriction to privileged
women. Only women of privilege, with enough to eat, easy access
to medical care, and the leisure to contemplate their "identity" are
attracted to "natural" childbirth.

As Johnson explains, "It is a rejection of privilege that simultaneously confirms it."

It is not surprising, then, that "natural" childbirth, a philosophy of privilege, is rejected by women who lack social privilege, women of color, and women from non-first-world countries. But there is a further reason for rejection, the romanticization of the experience of nonprivileged women:

> Third World women's experiences with traditional or natural birthing practices have been appropriated and romanticized by first world women, often to the detriment of the subaltern women.

To put it bluntly, privileged women construct a view of childbirth that explicitly ignores the vast suffering endured by real women forced to experience childbirth "naturally."

> The fantasy of Third World women's natural experiences of childbirth has become iconic among first world women, even if these experiences are more imagined than real. This creates multiple opportunities for exploitation, as the experiences of Third World women are used as a means for first world women to acquire knowledge, experience and perspective on "natural" or "traditional" birthing practices, while denying the importance of medical services that privileged women take for granted.

Natural childbirth is generally rejected by women of color and by women from countries outside the first world. Natural childbirth is a philosophy that presumes economic security, ready access to medical technology, and the leisure to construct an "identity." It does not merely ignore the difficulty that childbirth entails for many nonprivileged women, it actively erases their suffering by pretending that it does not exist and never existed.

NATURAL CHILDBIRTH ADVOCATES: WHITESPLAININ' BIRTH TO EVERYONE ELSE

According to Arthur Chu, in a brilliantly titled piece in the *Daily Beast*, "Who Died and Made You Khaleesi?":

> Mansplaining, whitesplaining, richsplaining—the way you can tell someone who's "privileged" is the unconscious belief that they have something to say, and that everyone will listen.[4]

Chu is not writing about natural parenting, but he could be:

> We repeatedly tell stories about a white protagonist who goes on a journey of self-discovery by mingling with exotic brown foreigners and becoming better at said foreigners' culture than they themselves are.

That accurately sums up natural parenting advocates' fantasy that they are emulating exotic brown foreigners and then becoming better at birth, breastfeeding, and parenting than those they were emulating.

Chu is brutally honest:

> The frustrating thing about being annoyed by the Mighty Whitey trope—and there are a ton of people

upset—is that it's so frequently employed by the well-meaning "good guys." The whole point of "going native" is that the familiar Western civilization is portrayed as inauthentic, ugly, broken, flawed. The "exotic" foreign civilization is somehow more natural, more primal, more sensual, the way people really ought to live.

That's a perfect characterization of the natural childbirth movement, complete with "Mighty Whiteys" like Grantly Dick-Read, who claimed that "primitive" women don't have pain in childbirth, or Ina May Gaskin, who is constantly invoking the supposed "sexuality" of birth in nature.

Why?

Is it just that we get sick of living in modern society with McDonald's and McMansions and mandatory vaccinations so we develop intricate fantasies about how much better life would be if we had to hunt our own food, build our own shelter, and develop our own resistance to dangerous microorganisms?

When it comes to natural parenting, the answer to that question is a resounding yes.

Natural childbirth is whitesplainin' at its most self-absorbed. Those who run the natural childbirth movement (as well as the lactivist movement and the attachment parenting movement) believe that they have something to say and other women ought to be grateful that they deign to share their "wisdom." They are forever bemoaning the high rate of black maternal mortality or the low rate of black breastfeeding while doing precisely nothing to ameliorate the root conditions that lead to poor outcomes for black mothers and babies.

At the heart of natural childbirth, from its inception to this day, is the elaborate, sexist, and racist fantasy that life would be so much better if we could just emulate our "primitive" ancestors—in other words, whitesplainin' at its finest.

HOW NATURAL CHILDBIRTH ADVOCATES EXPLOIT WOMEN OF COLOR

Grantly Dick-Read's racist trope, that primitive women don't have pain in childbirth, is alive and well among contemporary natural childbirth advocates, who pretend to themselves that they are reenacting childbirth among indigenous peoples. Their fantasy bears as much resemblance to childbirth in nature as a third-grade Thanksgiving play bears to the real relationship between the Pilgrims and the "uncivilized" Native Americans they came to displace.

But the racism at play in this context extends even further. Natural childbirth advocates are positively eager to use the misfortunes of women of color to advance their own privileged agenda. They delight in pointing to relatively high rates of perinatal and maternal mortality overall in the United States (as compared to other, "whiter" countries), yet ignore that they are primarily the result of appalling death rates among African-American women and their babies. Natural childbirth advocates and organizations have the unmitigated gall to imply that these women are dying of "too much" medical intervention when the reality is that they are dying of too little intervention for the serious complications many unfortunately face.

Ina May Gaskin, a privileged white woman, has led the way. She never misses an opportunity to highlight mortality rates and even created a "Safe Motherhood" quilt project[5] to draw attention to the problem. Gaskin represents herself as shocked at the current rate of maternal mortality. Yet as far as far as I can tell, home-birth midwives in general and Gaskin in particular have done nothing (no research, no education, no fundraising) to reduce the incidence of maternal mortality.

Anyone who visits the quilt website will notice something rather curious. There is no information about the causes, treatments, and research into maternal mortality. There are no scientific papers about maternal mortality. There is nothing about the epidemiology of maternal mortality. There is certainly no focus on the mortality of women and babies of color.

In my view, natural childbirth advocates only care about the deaths of women and babies of color only to the extent that they can exploit these for their own ends. The exploitation of women of color extends to the many ham-handed attempts to increase breastfeeding rates. For example, ending gifts of free formula samples does nothing to increase the rate of breastfeeding. Its only real impact is to deprive poor women (among which women of color are overrepresented) of a desperately needed resource for infant formula.

None of this is surprising. The natural childbirth movement is by, about, and for privileged white women. It rests to a large extent on misrepresenting women of color, while simultaneously exploiting the poor outcomes of those very same women in a thoroughly disingenuous critique of modern obstetrics.

It may be unconscious racism, but it is racism nonetheless.

BREASTFEEDING: HOW PRIVILEGED WOMEN MAKE PRIVILEGED CHOICES THE NORM

Lactivism, like natural childbirth and attachment parenting, is a philosophy of privilege.

Sociologist Orit Avishai explores this issue in the chapter "Managing the Lactating Body: The Breastfeeding Project in the Age of Anxiety."[6] Avishai immediately gets to the heart of the matter:

> Like other parenting, reproductive, health and lifestyle choices, breastfeeding is an option framed by access to resources, corporate interests, public policy, competing ideas about science, motherhood and standards of infant care. The construction of breastfeeding as a maternal project sheds light on breastfeeding disparities ("successful" breastfeeders tend to be white, educated, older and heterosexually partnered mothers) and on the fallacy of the "breast is best" and "breastfeeding is natural" slogans.

That goes a long way toward explaining why breastfeeding has been aggressively promoted in public health campaigns despite the fact that it has only trivial benefits. These campaigns have been motivated in large part by privileged white women reinscribing and reinforcing their privilege by declaring their personal preferences to be morally superior to those of poor women and women of color.

It is well established that breastfeeding rates differ markedly by race and class. As Avishai notes:

> [T]he "breast is best" frame creates a standard of good mothering that faults mothers who cannot comply with this standard or do not wish to comply with it. These mothers are usually poor, uneducated and minority women, some of whom resist what they see as imposition of white, middle-class mothering standards.

The heart of Avishai's argument is that, contrary to the claims of lactivists, breastfeeding as practiced in contemporary America is not natural. Indeed, the "lactating body [is] a carefully managed site and breastfeeding [is] a 'project'—a task to be researched, planned, implemented and assessed."

Breastfeeding as a project is promoted in part because of the commercialization of breastfeeding.

What does managing the lactating body involve? Avishai conducted in-depth interviews with first-time educated workforce-experienced and class-privileged mothers in the San Francisco Bay Area and created this list based on what she learned.

< Consulting books and asking experts
< Setting goals and assessing the product
< Managing the uncooperative lactating body
< Investing in production facilities

Each stage is mediated by privilege, and most require money. In contrast to the claims of lactivists, breastfeeding is no longer free.

Since the physiology of lactation assumes proper levels of nourishment and rest as well as maternal health—all stratified in the United States—the very construction of breast milk as "free" by mothers and lactation experts masks social inequalities. In addition . . . participants in my study embraced the expanding market of nursing gear, gadgets and accessories. They invested in nursing bras (around $40), nursing pads, breast pumps and related kits ($200–400), nursing pillows (around $40) and nursing chairs (around $200). Some purchased herbal supplements to enhance their milk supply or acquired breastfeeding outfits.

Breastfeeding is an expensive endeavor now, with many accoutrements that only the privileged can afford. Avishai concludes:

> Analysis of the mothering project sheds light on the obstacles encountered by women who cannot mobilise such resources, which are no longer considered optional. Viewed in this light, the twin constructs of "the breast is best" and "breastfeeding is natural" are impoverished slogans that do not capture the extent to which both the science and the imagery of breastfeeding are shaped by normative assumptions and middle-class experiences.

In other words, breastfeeding is a mark of race and class that provides marginal benefits but serves as a visible sign of privileged status.

WHEN LACTIVISTS LIE

Though she's hardly the first prominent person to lie in order to maintain her place in the natural parenting pantheon, blogger Jessica Martin-Weber of *The Leaky Boob* recently admitted that she lied about breastfeeding:

> I'm sorry that I've not been honest. . . .
> For every single one of my six beautiful children, bottles and breast have been a part of me reaching my goals. And not just because I had to go back to work. I choose to go back to work, I love working and am a

better parent when I work, but even when I didn't work outside the home, I elected to partially bottle feed my milk to my baby. This was a positive thing for me as I get physically stimulated very easily and as an introvert found the need to create some space for myself. I did better mentally and emotionally, which meant I was in a healthier place mentally and emotionally to parent my children. It was the best healthy choice for us.[7]

There are lots of problems with that lie, but one problem is bigger than all the others.

First the small problems:

1. *It is wrong to lie.* That pretty much goes without saying. Lying is not a good way to relate to others. It is a fundamental violation of their trust and has long-term consequences. People will be much less likely to trust you going forward.

2. *It is wrong to hold yourself out as a role model.* Our heroes have feet of clay; that's hardly news, but it is still disappointing. That's why anyone who presumes to hold herself out as a lactivist hero as Martin-Weber did should be very sure that she is modeling the behavior that she extols. Martin-Weber knew the entire time that she was presenting herself as a hero, she was actually engaging in the very behavior she was ostentatiously condemning in print.

3. *It is wrong to value process over outcome.* Of course this is standard operating procedure for natural childbirth advocates and lactivists. Instead of judging their mothering skills by how their children turn out (which raises the possibility that they might not end up being

declared perfect mothers), they evaluate their mothering skills by comparison with an arbitrary ideal. That way they can preen of their motherly perfection without the pesky need to wait until their children grow up and see how they turn out.

But most important:

4. The Leaky Boob's lie demonstrates that lactivism isn't about breastfeeding, and it isn't even about babies. It's about mothers and their own self-image.

Why was Jessica Martin-Weber writing about her breastfeeding experiences in the first place? It wasn't to benefit her children, since they couldn't care less how random strangers view their mother. And it wasn't to help other mothers with their breastfeeding difficulties, since Martin-Weber refused to be honest about her own.

Martin-Weber was writing (dishonestly) about her breastfeeding experiences in order to bask in the adulation of strangers and boost her own self-esteem. Breastfeeding isn't nearly so important to babies, but it is to lactivists.

So much of lactivism is about image, and new mothers would benefit greatly by realizing that. No mother should feel guilty about breastfeeding, because it is trivial in the overall scheme of child-rearing. Those who wish to convince you differently have their *own* best interests at heart, not yours and not your children's. In fact, they are so concerned about their own interests that they are willing to lie to maintain those interests.

NATURAL PARENTING AND SHOPPING YOUR WAY TO SAFETY

Many people have a need to signal their privileged status to others by adopting lifestyles and routines that require substantial steady incomes to support. It's pretty obvious when it comes to conspicuous consumption of expensive cars, designer clothes, and monstrously large homes. It is less obvious, though no less important, in natural and attachment parenting. It turns out to be very expensive to parent "naturally."

The concept of natural parenting as a visible marker of privilege raises an interesting and ironic possibility. Is natural parenting, often viewed as a rejection of contemporary consumer culture, merely a niche form of the very same consumer culture that is purportedly being rejected? In other words, just as the women who feed their children McDonald's takeout, let them play with plastic toys, and allow them to watch TV are obviously responding to rampant consumerism, are natural parenting advocates who hire doulas, treat everything with homeopathic remedies, and wear their babies in slings unwittingly responding to the exact same consumerism they claim to deplore, albeit consumerism carefully targeted specifically at them?

Is natural parenting about health, or is it just a giant marketing tactic created to sell worthless products? Do purveyors of natural parenting goods and service promote "shopping your way to safety"?

Rutgers sociologist Norah MacKendrick raises this disturbing possibility in her paper "More Work for Mother: Chemical Body Burdens as a Maternal Responsibility."[8] MacKendrick is writing specifically about preventing exposure to "toxins," but her observations apply to the wider world of natural parenting. MacKendrick firmly situates attachment parenting as a *consumer* choice:

The ideology of intensive mothering infuses spaces of consumption by urging mothers to buy with the best interests of the child in mind. Consumption is therefore entangled with other routine activities that parents—and mothers in particular—view as integral to securing a child's future outcomes. Indeed, women's transition to motherhood is marked by the consumption of specific material goods.

Mothers create elaborate rituals around shopping for and purchasing items that they believe are necessary to avoid "toxins." For example:

> Megan, a middle-class woman with an infant, has a complex precautionary consumption routine. . . . She consults books, magazines, and websites to find information about chemical avoidance and organizes her shopping list according to what items should be organic and nontoxic (e.g., meat, dairy, produce, cleaning products).

So Megan peruses magazines and websites (filled with ads for products she might purchase), then makes specific product choices in areas ranging from food to cleaning products. What's the difference between Megan and the woman who peruses *Vogue* and then makes specific product choices among designer options? Nothing, really.

And of course, like most natural parenting, the conspicuous consumption is traditionally gendered.

> Megan explains that her husband "is on board with it, but he definitely doesn't initiate. It just wouldn't enter

his realm of thought." When he does the grocery shopping, she "send[s] him out" with a list of specific brands of items to buy for their child, as she would not trust him to make the "right" choices.

Living a privileged life in a privileged neighborhood is almost a necessity:

Megan lives in a neighborhood with stores selling free-range chicken and discount organic foods. During our interview, she shows me a baby chair that she bought at a local store, and speaks enthusiastically about the natural wood and organic cotton.

Moreover, shopping your way to safety offers women an unmerited sense of superiority, as another mother demonstrates:

Cara considers precautionary consumption as an expression of vigilant mothering that protects against health problems: "I want it to be organic, to be as pure as possible—you know, they can put a lot of crazy ingredients in there . . . that's why all these kids are medicated, they're eating all this crappy stuff and then they can't behave themselves and what's it doing to them?"

While Megan and Cara claim, and probably even believe, that they are protecting their children's health by avoiding "toxins," they've actually been tricked into paying top dollar for products they likely don't need, don't make their children safer, advertise their privilege, and provide no additional value for the additional expense. They are no different from the less privileged women they look down upon for responding to the consumerist culture in which we live. They too have been manipulated into buying stuff in response to aggressive marketing campaigns, just different ones.

Similarly, natural parenting is not about the health and well-being of children. It's an industry with sophisticated marketing tactics designed to create and leverage maternal guilt in order to convince privileged women to buy an array of dubious products and services in an orgy of conspicuous consumption.

NEW MOTHERHOOD: THE LAST BASTION OF ACCEPTABLE BULLYING

We are all anti-bullying now.

We recognize that bullying based on race is wrong; bullying based on religion is wrong; bullying based on gender is wrong; bullying based on sexual orientation is wrong. In fact, there's only one group that it is still acceptable to bully: new mothers.

And who are the bullies? Lactivists, natural childbirth activists, and the natural parenting industry.

How do these activists and industries bully new mothers? Let me count the ways we've explored:

1. **The subversion of science.** From individual lactivists to the so-called Baby-Friendly Hospital Initiative, from individual birth bloggers to large organizations like Lamaze International and the Childbirth Connection, natural parenting advocates subvert the scientific evidence on breastfeeding and childbirth.

   The perversion of science is, if anything, even worse in natural childbirth advocacy. Childbirth with modern obstetrics is actually dramatically safer than natural childbirth. That hasn't stopped activists from lying about it. There is no lie that is too ridiculous for natural childbirth advocates to swallow: Michel Odent says pain is necessary for bonding; midwives promote "normal" birth as if the process is more important than the outcome; and there is no limit to the nonsense that issues forth from the mouths and pens of natural childbirth advocates (C-sections change DNA? C-sections destroy the infant microbiome?).

2. **Emotional abuse.** Among middle school girls, there is probably no insult more devastating than "no one likes you." That's why it is wielded so promiscuously among middle school bullies. Among new mothers, there is probably no insult more devastating than "your baby hasn't bonded to you." That's why lactivist and natural childbirth bullies wield it so promiscuously among new mothers. There is *no evidence* that bottle-fed babies are less bonded to their mothers than breastfed babies; there is *no evidence* that C-section babies are less bonded to their mothers than babies born by vaginal delivery. That hasn't stopped activists from repeatedly invoking bonding to force new mothers into compliance with the ethos of the group.

3. **Petty humiliations.**

"You only think you didn't produce enough milk for your baby."

"Your C-section was unnecessary."

"Bottle-feeding is so much easier; not surprising that you gave up breastfeeding and used formula instead."

Or the humble brag version: "I breastfeed because I'm lazy. Who wants to sterilize all those bottles?"

"What a shame that your baby was born drugged because you gave in and got an epidural."

4. **Institutional humiliations.** The Baby-Friendly Hospital Initiative has to be the biggest oxymoron in contemporary maternity care. This credentialing initiative isn't baby friendly and it certainly isn't mother friendly. It's bully friendly. It is based on the premise that any woman who doesn't wholeheartedly embrace breastfeeding must be forced to do so by constant hectoring, shaming, inconvenience (locking up formula), sleep deprivation (mandatory rooming in), and punishment (banning formula gifts).

I could go on, but I think you get the idea. Most of what passes for lactivism and natural childbirth advocacy is poorly disguised bullying.

Although we have gone a long way toward reducing bullying based on race, religion, gender, and sexual orientation, we have a long, long way to go. The tendency to bully appears to be innate to human beings; therefore, we must always be on guard against it.

Unfortunately, new motherhood appears to be the last bastion of acceptable bullying, where shaming, blaming, and humiliating new mothers has been sugar-coated as "science" and "education" when it is neither. It's just old-fashioned bullying, and the sooner we acknowledge that, the better.

Conclusion

Push Back Against the Guilt of Natural Parenting

Contrary to what the natural childbirth, lactivism, and attachment parenting movements would lead you to believe, being a good mother is about choosing mothering, not specific mothering choices. What does choosing mothering mean? It means actively embracing the role of caretaker, confidante, educator, and moral guide that mothering entails. It means worrying, planning, consulting, advising, and ultimately letting go of your children.

It is kissing the boo-boos, helping them face the fears, stepping aside, and allowing them to talk to the doctor in private when they are old enough. It is piano lessons, orthodontia, religious services, holiday celebrations. It is not responding when she says, "I hate you!" and never failing to respond when you see him teasing another child. It is hard, damn hard, with weeks or months that leave you exhausted or emotionally drained. Yet it is also rewarding at the deepest level, forging a bond to last a lifetime, launching a happy young adult into the world.

It is *not* about specific mothering choices. Breast or bottle? That's the mother's choice and nobody else's business. Natural childbirth? Irrelevant. Baby wearing? It depends on the baby and on the mother. Extended breastfeeding? Meaningless in the long run (and often in the short run, too).

The fundamental problem with the philosophies of natural childbirth, lactivism, and attachment parenting is not the emphasis that they place on mothering; it's the fact that they privilege specific mothering choices over others. In other words, adherents believe their own mothering choices proclaim their "goodness" and that different choices on the part of other mothers identify them as bad mothers.

Instead of viewing mothering as a service they willingly give their children, they view it as a social identity that they construct for themselves, boosting their own egos in the process. That's why discussions about natural childbirth, breastfeeding, and attachment parenting are such a source of discord between women. None of those discussions is about the best way to mother a baby; they're all about who is the best mother. It may seem like a trivial difference, but it is an immense difference, and most women recognize it as such. And the guilt that most mothers feel for not holding up to the irrational, unsound standards of the natural parenting movement is overwhelming and unnecessary.

The most critical ingredient of good mothering is love. A child who is loved has the advantage over any other child, regardless of the specific parenting choices his mother made. It's time to acknowledge and value the power of choosing motherhood, for women to stop judging other women based on mothering choices, and for mothers to stop judging themselves based on the personal preferences of a privileged few. It's time to push back, avoid the guilt trap, and embrace the enjoyment of motherhood.

Acknowledgments

Unlike my four children, whom my husband and I created with tools we had around the house, the completion of *Push Back* required the help of many friends and professionals.

I'd like to thank my brilliant agent, Gillian MacKenzie, who understood what I was trying to do and helped me do it, and editor Carrie Thornton, who shared my vision and saw it through to completion.

Thank you to Joan Liebmann-Smith, who helped me get started.

Thank you to the friends and colleagues who brainstormed with me and read parts of the manuscript: Dale Smith, Lori Lieberman, Nadine Tung, MD, Suzanne Barston, and Susan Lemagie, MD.

A special thank-you to the commenters on my blog, the smartest, wittiest, most articulate commenters on the Internet. I continue to learn from you each and every day and I cannot begin to express how much I value our virtual friendship.

Finally, I want to offer my deepest gratitude to the many women who, through private correspondence, have shared their anguish and guilt about childbirth, breastfeeding, and parenting travails. Some have given me permission to tell their stories in this volume, but there are many more whose stories could not be included for reasons of space. I am conscious of the honor that you have done me by confiding in me and I hope this book rewards your confidence in my ability to bear witness and to ease your pain.

Notes

CHAPTER 1. NATURAL CHILDBIRTH IS NOTHING LIKE CHILDBIRTH IN NATURE

1. Grantly Dick-Read. *Childbirth Without Fear*. New York: Harper & Bros, 1944.
2. Grantly Dick-Read. *Motherhood in the Post-War World*, London: Heinemann, 1944.
3. Grantly Dick-Read. *Revelation of Childbirth: The Principles and Practice of Natural Childbirth*. London: Heinemann Medical Books, 1942.
4. Paula A. Michaels. *Lamaze: An International History*. New York: Oxford University Press, 2014.
5. "Achievements in Public Health, 1900–1999: Healthier Mothers and Babies." Centers for Disease Control and Prevention, *MMWR Weekly*, October 1, 1999; cdc.gov/mmwr/preview/mmwrhtml/mm4838a2.htm.
6. Marlene Zuk. *Paleofantasy: What Evolution Really Tells Us About Sex, Diet, and How We Live*. New York: Norton, 2013.
7. Ina May Gaskin. *Ina May's Guide to Childbirth*. New York: Bantam, 2003.
8. K. C. Smith, A. S. Blunden, K. E. Whitwell, K. A. Dunn, and A. D. Wales. "A Survey of Equine Abortion, Stillbirth and Neonatal Death in the UK from 1988 to 1997." *Equine Veterinary Journal* 35.5 (2003): 496–501.
9. E. M. Huffman, J. H. Kirk, and M. Pappaioanou. "Factors Associated with Neonatal Lamb Mortality." *Theriogenology* 24, no. 2 (1985): 163–71.
10. R. Tønnessen, K. Sverdrup Borge, A. Nødtvedt, and A. Indrebø. "Canine Perinatal Mortality: A Cohort Study of 224 Breeds." *Theriogenology* 77.9 (2012): 1788–801.

11. Demography of Longevity. citeseerx.ist.psu.edu/viewdoc/download ?doi=10.1.1.513.1800&rep=rep1&type=pdf.

12. Sara Wickham. "Homebirth: What Are the Issues?" *Midwifery Today*, Summer 1999; midwiferytoday.com/articles/homebirthissues.asp.

13. "Miscarriage: MedlinePlus Medical Encyclopedia." US National Library of Medicine, November 8, 2012. Accessed April 19, 2015. nlm.nih.gov/medlineplus/ency/article/001488.htm.

14. Delores LaPratt. "Childbirth Prayers in Medieval and Early Modern England." *Symposia: The Graduate Student Journal of the Department for the Study of Religion at the University of Toronto* 2 (2010).

15. Judith Walzer Leavitt. "Under the Shadow of Maternity: American Women's Responses to Death and Debility Fears in Nineteenth-Century Childbirth." *Feminist Studies* 12, no. 1 (1986): 129–54.

16. "1 Million Babies Die the Day They're Born, Save the Children Says." Save the Children. N.p., n.d. Accessed April 8, 2015.

17. Jelka Zupan and Elisabeth Åhman. *Neonatal and Perinatal Mortality: Country, Regional and Global Estimates 2004.* Geneva: World Health Organization, 2007. Accessed December 14, 2015. apps.who.int/iris /bitstream/10665/43800/1/9789241596145_eng.pdf.

18. T. Lander. *Neonatal and Perinatal Mortality: Country, Regional and Global Estimates.* World Health Organization, 2006.

19. T. Kusiako, Carine Ronsmans, and L. Van der Paal. "Perinatal Mortality Attributable to Complications of Childbirth in Matlab, Bangladesh." *Bulletin of the World Health Organization* 78, no. 5 (2000): 621–27.

20. J. D. Ke. Ngowa, J. M. Kasia, A. Ekotarh, and C. Nzedjom. "Neonatal Outcome of Term Breech Births: A 15-Year Review at the Yaoundé General Hospital, Cameroon." *Clinics in Mother and Child Health* 9, no. 1 (2012).

21. A. Fong, C. T. Chau, D. Pan, and D. A. Ogunyemi. "Clinical Morbidities, Trends, and Demographics of Eclampsia: A Population-Based Study." *American Journal of Obstetrics and Gynecology* 209, no. 3 (2013): 229.

22. "Better Births." Royal College of Midwives. Accessed April 16, 2015. rcmnormalbirth.org.uk/.

23. Mary Ann Stark. "Preserving Normal Birth." *Journal of Obstetric, Gynecologic, & Neonatal Nursing* 37, no. 1 (2008): 84.

24. Beverley A. Lawrence Beech and Belinda Phipps. "Normal Birth: Women's Stories." *Normal Childbirth: Evidence and Debate*, 2nd ed., ed. Soo Downe. London: Churchill Livingstone Elsevier, 2008, p. 67.

25. Margaret E. MacDonald. "The Cultural Evolution of Natural Birth." *The Lancet* 378, no. 9789 (2011): 394–95.

26. "About Trust Birth," Trust Birth Initiative. Accessed April 9, 2013. trustbirth.com/about.html.

27. Sheena Byrom and Soo Downe. *The Roar Behind the Silence: Why Kindness, Compassion and Respect Matter in Maternity Care.* London: Pinter & Martin, 2015.

28. Gavin de Becker. *The Gift of Fear: Survival Signals That Protect Us from Violence.* Boston: Little, Brown, 1997.

CHAPTER 2. INTERVENTIONS ARE PREVENTIVE MEDICINE

1. "No Hatting, Patting or Chatting Class | Aamishop.com." Ancient Art of Midwifery Institute. Accessed April 16, 2015. 12.aamishop .com/nohats.html.

2. Judith A. Lothian, Debby Amis, and Jeannette Crenshaw. "Care Practice #4: No Routine Interventions." *The Journal of Perinatal Education* 16, no. 3 (2007): 29–34.

3. Henci Goer. *The Thinking Woman's Guide to a Better Birth.* New York: Perigee, 1999.

4. Zarko Alfirevic, Declan Devane, and G. M. Gyte. "Continuous Cardiotocography (CTG) As a Form of Electronic Fetal Monitoring (EFM) for Fetal Assessment During Labour." *Cochrane Database of Systematic Reviews* 3, no. 3 (2006): CD006066.

5. "PeriFACTS." PeriFACTS. Accessed April 16, 2015. perifacts.eu/ cases/Case_680_Fetal_Heart_Rate_Interpretation.php.

6. Han-Yang Chen, Suneet P. Chauhan, Cande V. Ananth, Anthony M. Vintzileos, and Alfred Z. Abuhamad. "Electronic Fetal Heart Rate Monitoring and Its Relationship to Neonatal and Infant Mortality in the United States." *American Journal of Obstetrics and Gynecology* 204, no. 6 (2011): 491-e1.

7. Harry Oxorn. *Human Labor and Birth*. Norwalk, CT: Appleton-Century-Crofts, 1986, p. 625.

8. F. Gary Cunningham et al. *Williams Obstetrics*, 22nd ed. New York: McGraw-Hill Professional, 2005, p. 535.

9. Ibid., p. 542.

10. M. F. MacDorman, S. E. Kirmeyer, and E. C. Wilson. "Fetal and Perinatal Mortality, United States, 2006." *National Vital Statistics Reports from the Centers for Disease Control and Prevention*, National Center for Health Statistics, National Vital Statistics System 60, no. 8 (2012): 1–22.

11. Sarah J. Stock, Evelyn Ferguson, Andrew Duffy, Ian Ford, James Chalmers, and Jane E. Norman. "Outcomes of Elective Induction of Labour Compared with Expectant Management: Population Based Study." *BMJ* 344 (2012): e2838.

12. Judith Lothian. "Saying 'No' to Induction." ncbi.nlm.nih.gov/pmc/articles/PMC1595289/.

13. MacDorman et al. "Fetal and Perinatal Mortality, United States, 2006."

14. Joyce A. Martin, Brady E. Hamilton, and Michelle J. K Osterman. "Births in the United States, 2013." *NCHS Data Brief* 175 (2014): 1–8.

15. Stock et al. "Outcomes of Elective Induction of Labour Compared with Expectant Management: Population Based Study."

16. Tamara Kaufman. "Evolution of the Birth Plan." *The Journal of Perinatal Education* 16, no. 3 (2007): 47.

17. Angela Pennell, Victoria Salo-Coombs, Amy Herring, Fred Spielman, and Karamarie Fecho. "Anesthesia and Analgesia-Related Preferences and Outcomes of Women Who Have Birth Plans." *Journal of Midwifery & Women's Health* 56, no. 4 (2011): 376–81.

18. Ingela Lundgren, Marie Berg, and Gunilla Lindmark. "Is the Childbirth Experience Improved by a Birth Plan?" *Journal of Midwifery & Women's Health* 48, no. 5 (2003): 322–28.

19. Ruth E. Gilbert and Pat A. Tookey. "Perinatal Mortality and Morbidity Among Babies Delivered in Water: Surveillance Study and Postal Survey." *BMJ* 319, no. 7208 (1999): 483–87.

20. "Waterbirth FAQ." Waterbirth FAQ. Accessed November 30, 2015. waterbirth.org/index.php?option=com_content&view=article&id=69.

21. A. Thoeni, N. Zech, L. Moroder, and F. Ploner. "Review of 1600 Water Births. Does Water Birth Increase the Risk of Neonatal Infection?" *Journal of Maternal-Fetal and Neonatal Medicine* 17, no. 5 (2005): 357–61.

22. "Linked Birth / Infant Death Records, 2007–2013 Request." Accessed December 01, 2015. wonder.cdc.gov/lbd-current.html.

23. "2011 CO Midwifery Statistical Summary.pdf." Google Docs. Accessed December 1, 2015. drive.google.com/file/d/0B-K5DhxXx JZbSExoRWJ2S1o3cUU/view.

24. California Licensed Midwife Annual Report Summary, and page 1 of 7, *California Licensed Midwife Annual Report Summary*. Accessed December 1, 2015. mbc.ca.gov/Licensees/Midwives/mid wives_2010_annual_report.pdf.

25. Judith Rooks, CNM. March 15, 2013. Accessed December 1, 2015. olis.leg.state.or.us/liz/2013R1/Downloads/CommitteeMeetingDoc ument/8585.

26. "Data and Statistics." Centers for Disease Control and Prevention. October 22, 2015. Accessed December 1, 2015. cdc.gov/sids/data.htm.

27. Melissa Cheyney, Marit Bovbjerg, Courtney Everson, Wendy Gordon, Darcy Hannibal, and Saraswathi Vedam. "Outcomes of Care for 16,924 Planned Home Births in the United States: The Midwives Alliance of North America Statistics Project, 2004 to 2009." *Journal of Midwifery & Women's Health* 59, no. 1 (2014): 17–27.

28. S. E. Buitendijk and J. G. Nijhuis. "High Perinatal Mortality in the Netherlands Compared to the Rest of Europe." *Nederlands tijdschrift voor geneeskunde* 148, no. 38 (2004): 1855–60.

CHAPTER 3. THERE IS NO BENEFIT TO REFUSING PAIN RELIEF

1. "Women Who Have Caesareans 'Less Likely to Bond.'" *Mail Online*, July 13, 2006. Accessed April 17, 2015. dailymail.co.uk/health/article -395218/Women-Caesareans-likely-bond.html.

2. Karen R. Rosenberg and Wenda R. Trevathan. "The Evolution of Human Birth." *Scientific American* 13 (2003): 80–85.

3. Maya Suresh, Roanne L. Preston, Roshan Fernando, and M. D. C LaToya Mason. *Shnider and Levinson's Anesthesia for Obstetrics*. Baltimore, MD: Lippincott Williams & Wilkins, 2013, p. 155.

4. Ibid.

5. F. Gary Cunningham et al. *Williams Obstetrics*, 22nd ed. New York: McGraw-Hill Professional, 2005, p. 477.

6. Ibid., pp. 483–84.

7. Ibid., pp. 481–82.

8. JaneMaree Maher. "The Painful Truth About Childbirth: Contemporary Discourses of Caesareans, Risk and the Realities of Pain." tasa .org.au/conferences/conferencepapers07/papers/19.pdf.

9. Millicent Anim-Somuah, Rebecca Smyth, and Leanne Jones. "Epidural Versus Non-Epidural or No Analgesia in Labour." *Cochrane Database of Systematic Reviews* (2011).

10. Ban Leong Sng, Wan Ling Leong, Yanzhi Zeng, Fahad Javaid Siddiqui, Pryseley N. Assam, Yvonne Lim, Edwin S.Y. Chan, and Alex T. Sia. "Early Versus Late Initiation of Epidural Analgesia for Labour." *Cochrane Database of Systematic Reviews* (2014).

11. Henci Goer. "Epidurals: Do They or Don't They Increase Cesareans?" *Science & Sensibility*. Accessed December 1, 2015. scienceandsensibil ity.org/epidurals-do-they-or-dont-they-increase-cesareans/.

12. Judy Slome Cohain. "The Epidural Trip: Why Are So Many Women Taking Dangerous Drugs During Labor?" *Midwifery Today with International Midwife* 95 (2009): 21–4.

13. "Women Who Have Caesareans 'Less Likely to Bond.'"

14. "Pitocin—FDA Prescribing Information." Drug.com. Accessed April 17, 2015. drugs.com/pro/pitocin.html.

15. Judith A. Lothian. "The Birth of a Breastfeeding Baby and Mother." *Journal of Perinatal Education* 14, no. 1 (2005): 42.

16. "New Lamaze International Epidural Infographic—Information, Not Judgment." *Science & Sensibility*. Accessed December 1, 2015. science andsensibility.org/new-lamaze-international-epidural-infographic -information-not-judgment/.

17. "A Look at the Research: The Link Between Epidural Analgesia and Breastfeeding." *Science & Sensibility*, June 21, 2011. Accessed

April 17, 2015. scienceandsensibility.org/a-look-at-the-research-the
-link-between-epidural-analgesia-and-breastfeeding/.

18. Ashley L. Szabo. "Intrapartum Neuraxial Analgesia and Breastfeeding Outcomes: Limitations of Current Knowledge." *Anesthesia &
Analgesia* 116, no. 2 (2013): 399–405.

19. "Orgasmic Birth—The Best-Kept Secret." Orgasmic Birth. Accessed
April 17, 2015. orgasmicbirth.com/.

20. Jane Pincus. "Orgasmic Birth: The Best-Kept Secret." *Birth* 36, no. 3
(2009): 265–66.

21. "Childbirth Orgasms? Some Women Are Able to Experience Ecstatic
Birth [VIDEO]." *Medical Daily.* June 03, 2013. Accessed April 17,
2015. medicaldaily.com/childbirth-orgasms-some-women-are-able
-experience-ecstatic-birth-video-246468.

22. Ina May Gaskin. *Ina May's Guide to Childbirth.* New York: Bantam,
2008, xiii.

23. Ina May Gaskin. *Spiritual Midwifery.* Summertown, TN: Book Publications, 2002.

24. Helena Vissing. "Triumphing Over the Body: Body Fantasies and
Their Protective Functions." Accessed December 1, 2015. inter-dis
ciplinary.net/probing-the-boundaries/wp-content/uploads/2013/04
/hvissing_br1_wpaper.pdf.

CHAPTER 4. THE RIGHT C-SECTION RATE

1. F. Gary Cunningham et al. *Williams Obstetrics*, 22nd ed. New York:
McGraw-Hill Professional, 2005, p. 588.

2. Ibid., p. 503.

3. Ibid., p. 568.

4. Ibid., p. 591.

5. Marian F. MacDorman, Donna L. Hoyert, and T. J. Mathews.
"Recent Declines in Infant Mortality in the United States, 2005–
2011." *NCHS Data Brief* 120 (2013): 1–8.

6. Jennifer Block. "The C-section Epidemic." *Los Angeles Times.* September 24, 2007. Accessed April 17, 2015. latimes.com/news/la-oe
-block24sep24-story.html.

7. Paul Root Wolpe. "The Holistic Heresy: Strategies of Ideological

Challenge in the Medical Profession." *Social Science & Medicine* 31, no. 8 (1990): 913–23.

8. Steven L. Clark, Michael A. Belfort, Gary A. Dildy, Melissa A. Herbst, Janet A. Meyers, and Gary D. Hankins. "Maternal Death in the 21st Century: Causes, Prevention, and Relationship to Cesarean Delivery." *American Journal of Obstetrics and Gynecology* 199, no. 1 (2008): 36-e1.

9. Ibid.

10. Tamisha F. Johnson and Candace Mulready-Ward. "Pregnancy-Related Mortality in the United States, 1998 to 2005." *Obstetrics & Gynecology* 117, no. 5 (2011): 1229–30.

11. "Women Who Have Caesareans 'Less Likely to Bond.'" *Mail Online*, July 13, 2006. Accessed April 17, 2015. dailymail.co.uk/health/article -395218/Women-Caesareans-likely-bond.html.

12. World Health Organization, "Appropriate Technology for Birth." *The Lancet* 2 (1985): 436–37.

13. World Health Organization, UNFPA, UNICEF, and AMDD. "Monitoring Emergency Obstetric Care: A Handbook." Geneva: WHO, 2009.

14. Ana P. Betrán, Mario Merialdi, Jeremy A. Lauer, Wang Bing-Shun, Jane Thomas, Paul Van Look, and Marsden Wagner. "Rates of Caesarean Section: Analysis of Global, Regional and National Estimates." *Paediatric and Perinatal Epidemiology* 21, no. 2 (2007): 98–113.

15. "Epigenetics: Fundamentals." What Is Epigenetics. Accessed April 17, 2015. whatisepigenetics.com/fundamentals/.

16. Gunnar Kaati, Lars Olov Bygren, Marcus Pembrey, and Michael Sjöström. "Transgenerational Response to Nutrition, Early Life Circumstances and Longevity." *European Journal of Human Genetics* 15, no. 7 (2007): 784–90.

17. Malin Almgren, Titus Schlinzig, David Gomez-Cabrero, Agneta Gunnar, Mikael Sundin, Stefan Johansson, Mikael Norman, and Tomas J. Ekström. "Cesarean Delivery and Hematopoietic Stem Cell Epigenetics in the Newborn Infant: Implications for Future Health?" *American Journal of Obstetrics and Gynecology* 211, no. 5 (2014): 502-e1.

18. "UBC Midwifery to Welcome Prof. Soo Downe as the First Elaine Carty Visiting Scholar." Midwifery Program. Accessed December 01, 2015. midwifery.ubc.ca/2015/02/17/ubc-midwifery -to-welcome-prof-soo-downe-as-the-first-2015-elaine-carty -visiting-scholar/.

19. "The Epigenetic Jury Is Still Out on C-sections." Scienceline. June 12, 2012. Accessed April 17, 2015. http://scienceline.org/2012/06/the -epigenetic-jury-is-still-out-on-c-sections/.

20. Ibid.

21. "Microbirth." One World Birth. January 28, 2014. Accessed April 17, 2015. oneworldbirth.net/blog/the-end-of-our-journey/.

22. "FAQ: Human Microbiome, January 2014." American Society for Microbiology. January 2014. Accessed April 17, 2015. academy.asm .org/index.php/faq-series/5122-humanmicrobiome.

23. Cunningham. *Williams Obstetrics,* 608.

24. Mark B. Landon, Sharon Leindecker, Catherine Y. Spong, John C. Hauth, Steven Bloom, Michael W. Varner, Atef H. Moawad et al. "The MFMU Cesarean Registry: Factors Affecting the Success of Trial of Labor after Previous Cesarean Delivery." *American Journal of Obstetrics and Gynecology* 193, no. 3 (2005): 1016–23.

25. Cunningham. *Williams Obstetrics,* 608.

26. "ACOG Practice Bulletin: Vaginal Birth after Previous Cesarean Delivery. Number 2, October 1998. Clinical Management Guidelines for Obstetrician-Gynecologists." *International Journal of Gynaecology & Obstetrics* 64, no. 2 (1999): 201–08.

27. "Advocacy." International Cesarean Awareness Network. Accessed April 17, 2015. ican-online.org/advocacy/.

28. Landon et al. "The MFMU Cesarean Registry."

29. Ibid.

30. Mohammed A. Elkousy, Mary Sammel, Erika Stevens, Jeffrey F. Peipert, and George Macones. "The Effect of Birth Weight on Vaginal Birth after Cesarean Delivery Success Rates." *American Journal of Obstetrics and Gynecology* 188, no. 3 (2003): 824–30.

31. Kimberly D. Gregory, Lisa M. Korst, Moshe Fridman, Ida Shihady, Paula Broussard, Arlene Fink, and Linda Burnes Bolton. "Vaginal

Birth after Cesarean: Clinical Risk Factors Associated with Adverse Outcome." *American Journal of Obstetrics and Gynecology* 198, no. 4 (2008): 452-e1.

32. Celeste P. Durnwald, Hugh M. Ehrenberg, and Brian M. Mercer. "The Impact of Maternal Obesity and Weight Gain on Vaginal Birth after Cesarean Section Success." *American Journal of Obstetrics and Gynecology* 191, no. 3 (2004): 954–57.

33. Mark B. Landon, John C. Hauth, Kenneth J. Leveno, Catherine Y. Spong, Sharon Leindecker, Michael W. Varner, Atef H. Moawad et al. "Maternal and Perinatal Outcomes Associated with a Trial of Labor after Prior Cesarean Delivery." *New England Journal of Medicine* 351, no. 25 (2004): 2581–89.

34. David M. Stamilio, Emily DeFranco, Emmanuelle Paré, Anthony O. Odibo, Jeffrey F. Peipert, Jenifer E. Allsworth, Erika Stevens, and George A. Macones. "Short Interpregnancy Interval: Risk of Uterine Rupture and Complications of Vaginal Birth after Cesarean Delivery." *Obstetrics & Gynecology* 110, no. 5 (2007): 1075–82.

35. Anthony C. Sciscione, Mark B. Landon, Kenneth J. Leveno, Catherine Y. Spong, Cora MacPherson, Michael W. Varner, Dwight J. Rouse et al. "Previous Preterm Cesarean Delivery and Risk of Subsequent Uterine Rupture." *Obstetrics & Gynecology* 111, no. 3 (2008): 648–53.

36. "Why Kate Lied about Mia's Birth." *Mail Online*. Accessed April 17, 2015. dailymail.co.uk/tvshowbiz/article-300032/Why-Kate-lied-Mias-birth.html.

CHAPTER 5. BREAST IS *NOT* ALWAYS BEST

1. "Can Breastfeeding Prevent Illnesses?" LLLI. Accessed December 2, 2015. llli.org/faq/prevention.html.

2. Melissa Bartick and Arnold Reinhold. "The Burden of Suboptimal Breastfeeding in the United States: A Pediatric Cost Analysis." *Pediatrics* 125, no. 5 (2010): e1048–56.

3. "Importance of Breastfeeding." Baby-Friendly USA. Accessed

December 2, 2015. babyfriendlyusa.org/faqs/importance-of-breast feeding.

4. Michael S. Kramer, Beverley Chalmers, Ellen D. Hodnett, Zinaida Sevkovskaya, Irina Dzikovich, Stanley Shapiro, Jean-Paul Collet et al. "Promotion of Breastfeeding Intervention Trial (PROBIT): A Randomized Trial in the Republic of Belarus." *JAMA* 285, no. 4 (2001): 413–20.

5. Bernardo L. Horta and Cesar G. Victora. "Long-Term Effects of Breastfeeding: A Systematic Review." World Health Organization, 2013. who.int/maternal_child_adolescent/documents/breastfeeding _long_term_effects/en/.

6. Cynthia G. Colen and David M. Ramey. "Is Breast Truly Best? Estimating the Effects of Breastfeeding on Long-Term Child Health and Wellbeing in the United States Using Sibling Comparisons." *Social Science & Medicine* 109 (2014): 55–65.

7. Ruowei Li, Natalie Darling, Emmanuel Maurice, Lawrence Barker, and Laurence M. Grummer-Strawn. "Breastfeeding Rates in the United States by Characteristics of the Child, Mother, or Family: The 2002 National Immunization Survey." *Pediatrics* 115, no. 1 (2005): e31–37.

8. Philippe Van de Perre. "Transfer of Antibody via Mother's Milk." *Vaccine* 21, no. 24 (2003): 3374–76.

9. Angela Garbes. "The More I Learn About Breast Milk, the More Amazed I Am." *The Stranger*, August 26, 2015. Accessed December 2, 2015. thestranger.com/features/feature/2015/08/26/22755273/ the-more-i-learn-about-breast-milk-the-more-amazed-i-am.

10. Colen and Ramey. "Is Breast Truly Best?"

11. World Health Organization. "Long-Term Effects of Breastfeeding: A Systematic Review." Geneva: World Health Organization, 2013.

12. Valerie J. Flaherman, Janelle Aby, Anthony E. Burgos, Kathryn A. Lee, Michael D. Cabana, and Thomas B. Newman. "Effect of Early Limited Formula on Duration and Exclusivity of Breastfeeding in At-Risk Infants: An RCT." *Pediatrics* 131, no. 6 (2013): 1059–65.

13. Lawrence Noble. "What's Really Wrong with One Bottle: Micro-

biota & Metabolic Syndrome." May 13, 2014. misn-ny.org/documents /MidHudsonOneBottleTalkrev.pdf.

14. Jennifer Hahn-Holbrook, Chris Dunkel Schetter, and Martie Haselton. "Breastfeeding and Maternal Mental and Physical Health," in *Women's Health Psychology,* eds. Mary Spiers, Pamela Geller, and Jacqueline D. Kloss. New York: Wiley, 2013.

15. Joan B. Wolf. "Is Breast Really Best? Risk and Total Motherhood in the National Breastfeeding Awareness Campaign." *Journal of Health Politics, Policy and Law* 32, no. 4 (2007): 595–636.

16. Joan B. Wolf. *Is Breast Best? Taking on the Breastfeeding Experts and the New High Stakes of Motherhood.* New York: New York University Press, 2011.

17. Hanna Rosin. "The Case Against Breast-Feeding." *The Atlantic,* April 01, 2009. Accessed December 02, 2015. theatlantic.com/maga zine/archive/2009/04/the-case-against-breast-feeding/307311/.

18. Judith Graham. "Science Supports Breast-feeding but It's a Woman's Choice." *Triage.* April 3, 2009. Accessed December 2, 2015. news blogs.chicagotribune.com/triage/2009/04/tscience-supports-breast feeding-but-its-a-womans-choice.html.

19. Jennifer Block. "The Breastfeeding Fight for Baby Nutrition." *Babble,* April 20, 2009. Accessed December 2, 2015. babble.com/baby/the -breastfeeding-fight-for-baby-nutrition/.

20. Centers for Disease Control and Prevention (CDC). "Breastfeeding Report Card 2013, United States." Retrieved November 20, 2013.

21. Nancy M. Hurst. "Recognizing and Treating Delayed or Failed Lactogenesis II." *Journal of Midwifery & Women's Health* 52, no. 6 (2007): 588–94.

22. Charles Hirschman and Marilyn Butler. "Trends and Differentials in Breast Feeding: An Update." *Demography* 18, no. 1 (1981): 39–54.

23. Jack Newman. "Myths of Breastfeeding." Accessed December 2, 2015. nbci.ca/index.php?option=com_content&id=27%3Amyths-of -breastfeeding.

24. Jack Newman. "Protocol to Manage Breastmilk Intake." Accessed

December 2, 2015. breastfeedinginc.ca/content.php?pagename=doc +PMBI.

25. Jack Newman. "Facebook." Dr. Jack Newman. October 11, 2013. Accessed December 2, 2015. facebook.com/DrJackNewman/posts /243007675850286.

26. "Myopia (Nearsightedness)." American Optometric Association. Accessed April 17, 2015. aoa.org/patients-and-public/eye-and-vision -problems/glossary-of-eye-and-vision-conditions/myopia?sso=y.

27. "The Ten Steps to Successful Breastfeeding." Baby-Friendly USA. Accessed December 2, 2015. babyfriendlyusa.org/about-us/baby -friendly-hospital-initiative/the-ten-steps.

28. Mary Kay Linge. "Mayor Bloomberg Pushing NYC Hospitals to Hide Baby Formula so More New Moms Will Breast-Feed." *New York Post,* July 29, 2012. Accessed April 17, 2015. nypost.com/2012/07/29 /mayor-bloomberg-pushing-nyc-hospitals-to-hide-baby-formula-so -more-new-moms-will-breast-feed/.

29. Mark B. Cope and David B. Allison. "White Hat Bias: Examples of Its Presence in Obesity Research and a Call for Renewed Commit-ment to Faithfulness in Research Reporting." *International Journal of Obesity* 34, no. 1 (2010): 84–88.

30. Suzanne Michaels Cobb-Barston. *Bottled Up: How the Way We Feed Babies Has Come to Define Motherhood, and Why It Shouldn't.* Berkeley: University of California Press, 2012.

31. Anne L. Wright and Richard J. Schanler. "The Resurgence of Breast-feeding at the End of the Second Millennium." *Journal of Nutrition* 131, no. 2 (2001): 421S–425S.

32. James R. Flynn. *What Is Intelligence?: Beyond the Flynn Effect.* New York: Cambridge University Press, 2007.

33. Diane Wiessinger. "Watch Your Language." *Journal of Human Lacta-tion* 12, no. 1 (1996): 1–4.

34. Gill Thomson, Katherine Ebisch-Burton, and Renee Flacking. "Shame If You Do—Shame If You Don't: Women's Experiences of Infant Feeding." *Maternal & Child Nutrition* 11, no. 1 (2015): 33–46.

35. Emily Wax-Thibodeaux. "Why I Don't Breast-feed, If You Must

Know." *Washington Post*, October 13, 2014. Accessed April 17, 2015. washingtonpost.com/national/health-science/why-i-dont-breastfeed -if-you-must-know/2014/10/13/74c5fd3e-459a-11e4-9a15-137aa01 53527_story.html.

CHAPTER 6. NO SCIENCE SUPPORTS ATTACHMENT PARENTING

1. Sharon Hays. *The Cultural Contradictions of Motherhood*. New Haven, CT: Yale University Press, 1996.
2. Charlotte Faircloth. "Intensive Parenting and the Expansion of Parenting," in *Parenting Culture Studies*, eds. Ellie Lee, Jennie Bristow, Charlotte Faircloth, and Jan Macvarish. Houndmills, Basingstoke, Hampshire: Palgrave Macmillan, 2014, pp. 25–50.
3. William Sears and Martha Sears. *The Complete Book of Christian Parenting and Child Care: A Medical and Moral Guide to Raising Happy Healthy Children*. Nashville: B&H Books, 1997.
4. Faircloth. "Intensive Parenting and the Expansion of Parenting."
5. David Lancy. "Detachment Parenting." *Psychology Today,* February 17, 2012. psychologytoday.com/blog/benign-neglect/201202/de tachment-parenting.
6. "What Is Attachment Parenting?" Attachment Parenting International. Accessed April 17, 2015. attachmentparenting.org/WhatIsAP.php.
7. "John Bowlby." Wikipedia. Accessed April 28, 2015. en.wikipedia.org /wiki/John_Bowlby.
8. "Donald Winnicott." Wikipedia. Accessed April 28, 2015. en.wikipe dia.org/wiki/Donald_Winnicott.
9. "Harry Harlow." Wikipedia. Accessed April 28, 2015. en.wikipedia .org/wiki/Harry_Harlow.
10. Ibid.
11. William Sears and Martha Sears. *The Attachment Parenting Book: A Commonsense Guide to Understanding and Nurturing Your Baby*. Boston: Little, Brown, 2001.
12. "Infants & Toddlers." Accessed December 02, 2015. attachmentpar enting.org/parentingtopics/infants-toddlers.
13. Rebecca Kukla. *Mass Hysteria: Medicine, Culture, and Mothers' Bodies*. Lanham, MD: Rowman & Littlefield, 2005.

14. Kathryn M. Rizzo, Holly H. Schiffrin, and Miriam Liss. "Insight into the Parenthood Paradox: Mental Health Outcomes of Intensive Mothering." *Journal of Child and Family Studies* 22, no. 5 (2013): 614–20.

15. Avital Norman Nathman. "Do Ideal Images of Motherhood Impact Postpartum Depression?" *SheKnows,* February 13, 2015. sheknows .com/parenting/articles/1069807/do-ideal-images-of-motherhood -impact-postpartum-depression.

16. "Behind the Cover: Are You Mom Enough?" *Time*, May 10, 2012. Accessed April 17, 2015. time.com/3450144/behind-the-cover-are -you-mom-enough/.

17. Phyllis L. F. Rippeyoung. "Governing Motherhood: Who Pays and Who Profits." In Focus, Canadian Centre for Policy Alternatives, January 2013. policyalternatives.ca/publications/reports/governing -motherhood.

18. Susan Dominus. "Motherhood, Screened Off." *New York Times.* September 23, 2015. nytimes.com/2015/09/24/magazine/motherhood -screened-off.html?_r=1.

CHAPTER 7. WHO HIJACKED CHILDBIRTH?

1. "History of Midwifery." Dimensions Healthcare System. Accessed December 02, 2015. dimensionshealth.org/index.php/dimensions -health-services-prince-georges-county-maryland-md/midwifery/his tory-of-midwifery/.

2. Cara Kinzelman and Jesse Bushman. "Understanding Your Practice Environment." Accessed December 2, 2015. midwife.org/acnm/files /ccLibraryFiles/Filename/000000004315/Understanding-Practice -Environment.pdf.

3. Ibid.

4. Ellen Annandale and Judith Clark. "What Is Gender? Feminist Theory and the Sociology of Human Reproduction." *Sociology of Health & Illness* 18, no. 1 (1996): 17–44.

5. "Sheila Kitzinger." Wikipedia. Accessed December 02, 2015. en.wikipedia.org/wiki/Sheila_Kitzinger.

6. Robbie E. Davis-Floyd. *Birth As an American Rite of Passage*. Berkeley: University of California Press, 1992.

7. Henci Goer and Amy Romano. *Optimal Care in Childbirth: The Case for a Physiologic Approach*. Seattle: Classic Day Publishing, 2012.

8. "Ina May Gaskin." Wikipedia. Accessed December 02, 2015. en .wikipedia.org/wiki/Ina_May_Gaskin.

9. Jennifer A. Parratt and Kathleen M. Fahy. "Including the Nonrational Is Sensible Midwifery." *Women and Birth* 21, no. 1 (2008): 37–42.

10. Robbie Davis-Floyd. "The Technocratic Model of Birth." Accessed December 2, 2015. davis-floyd.com/uncategorized/the-technocratic -model-of-birth/.

11. Henci Goer. *The Thinking Woman's Guide to a Better Birth*. New York: Perigee Books, 1999.

12. Caroline H. Bledsoe and Rachel F. Scherrer. "The Dialectics of Disruption: Paradoxes of Nature and Professionalism in Contemporary American Childbearing." *Reproductive Disruptions: Gender, Technology, and Biopolitics in the New Millennium*, ed. Marcia C. Inhorn. New York: Berghahn Books, 2007, pp. 47–78.

13. Paula A. Michaels. *Lamaze: An International History*. New York: Oxford University Press, 2014, p. 149.

14. Charlotte A. De Vries and Raymond G. De Vries. "Childbirth Education in the 21st Century: An Immodest Proposal." *Journal of Perinatal Education* 16, no. 4 (2007): 38.

15. Susan Downe, ed. *Normal Childbirth: Evidence and Debate*. London: Churchill Livingstone Elsevier, 2008.

16. De Vries and De Vries. "Childbirth Education in the 21st Century."

17. Bill Kirkup. "The Report of the Morecambe Bay Investigation." March 2015. gov.uk/government/uploads/system/uploads/attachment _data/file/408480/47487_MBI_Accessible_v0.1.pdf.

18. Marie Hastings-Tolsma and Anna G. W. Nolte. "Reconceptualising Failure to Rescue in Midwifery: A Concept Analysis." *Midwifery* 30, no. 6 (2014): 585–94.

19. Daniel Martin. "Why Mothers Should Put Up with Pain of Childbirth—by a Male Expert in Midwifery." *Mail Online*, July 13, 2009. Accessed December 2, 2015. dailymail.co.uk/health /article-1199156/Why-mothers-pain-childbirth—male-expert-mid wifery.html#ixzz0LFdZkJbp&D.

20. Annandale and Clark. "What Is Gender?"

21. Barbara Katz Rothman. "Birth Junkies: Working Through Our Relationship to Birth," lecture, Midwives Alliance of North America Conference, 2008.

22. "Birth Doula Steps to DONA International Certification." *DONA International*, September 2014. Accessed April 18, 2015. http://www .dona.org/PDF/Birth+Doula_steps+to+cert_website_07-13.pdf.

23. "Traditional Childbirth Educator Certification." International Child birth Education Association. Accessed April 18, 2015. icea.org/con tent/traditional-childbirth-educator-certification.

24. "Doula." The Free Dictionary. Accessed April 17, 2015. thefreedictio nary.com/doula.

25. "Dona International's Impressive Growth." DONA. Accessed December 2, 2015. dona.org/aboutus/statistics.php.

26. "Annual Report 2014." Lamaze International. Accessed April 20, 2015. http% 3A%2F%2Fwww.lamazeinternational.org%2Fd%2Fdo %2F1587.

27. Abigail Locke and Mary Horton-Salway. "'Golden Age' Versus 'Bad Old Days': A Discursive Examination of Advice Giving in Antenatal Classes." *Journal of Health Psychology* 15, no. 8 (2010): 1214–24.

CHAPTER 8. THE COMMODIFICATION OF BIRTH

1. M. Rutherford & S. Gallo-Cruz. *Great Expectations: Emotion as Central to the Experiential Consumption of Birth.* Boston, MA: American Sociological Association, 2008.

2. Melanie Springer Mock. "Celebrating the Stories That Make Us Real by Melanie Springer Mock—1." *The Mothers Movement Online.* Accessed December 2, 2015. mothersmovement.org/features/07/03 /mock_1.html.

3. Pru Hobson-West. "'Trusting Blindly Can Be the Biggest Risk of All': Organised Resistance to Childhood Vaccination in the UK." *Sociology of Health & Illness* 29, no. 2 (2007): 198–215.

4. "The Story of Geneva's Birth—an HBC Journey." Homebirth Cesarean. April 21, 2014. homebirthcesarean.org/the-story-of-genevas -birth-an-hbc-journey/.

CHAPTER 9. THE BUSINESS OF BREASTFEEDING

1. Rima D. Apple. *Mothers and Medicine: A Social History of Infant Feeding, 1890–1950*, Wisconsin Publications in the History of Science and Medicine. Madison: University of Wisconsin Press, 1987.

2. Jacqueline H. Wolf. "Saving Babies and Mothers: Pioneering Efforts to Decrease Infant and Maternal Mortality." *Silent Victories: The History and Practice of Public Health in Twentieth-Century America,* ed. John Ward and Christian Warren. New York: Oxford University Press, 2006, 135.

3. Jule DeJager Ward. *La Leche League: At the Crossroads of Medicine, Feminism, and Religion.* Chapel Hill: University of North Carolina Press, 2000.

4. Ibid.

5. "A Brief History of La Leche League International." LLLI. July 27, 2012. Accessed April 18, 2015. llli.org/lllihistory.html?m=1 percent2 C0percent2C0.

6. "The LLL Leader and the IBCLC—A Partnership in Breastfeeding History." LLLI. June/July 2000. Accessed April 18, 2015. lalechelea gue.org/lllleaderweb/lv/lvjunjul00p52.html.

7. Harmony Danyelle Newman. "Cross-Cultural Framing Strategies of the Breastfeeding Movement and Mothers' Responses." PhD dissertation, Vanderbilt University, May 2010. etd.library.vanderbilt .edu/available/etd-02172010-152111/unrestricted/NewmanDisserta tionFinal.pdf

8. "Baby-Friendly Hospital Initiative." Baby-Friendly USA. Accessed April 17, 2015. babyfriendlyusa.org/about-us/baby-friendly-hospital -initiative.

9. "Breastfeeding." WHO. Accessed April 18, 2015. who.int/maternal _child_adolescent/topics/child/nutrition/breastfeeding/en/.

10. "Baby-Friendly Hospital Initiative."

11. "Baby-Friendly USA, Inc. Fee Schedule." Baby-Friendly USA, Inc., May 1, 2014. Accessed April 18, 2015. d14abeop4cfxkt.cloudfront .net/cms/files/295/files/original/Fee_Schedule_4-D_Pathway_Effec tive_7_1_14.pdf.

12. M. J. Renfrew, H. Spiby, L. D'Souza, L. M. Wallace, L. Dyson, and F. McCormick. "Rethinking Research in Breast-Feeding: A Critique of the Evidence Base Identified in a Systematic Review of Interventions to Promote and Support Breast-Feeding." *Public Health Nutrition* 10, no. 7 (2007): 726–32.

13. B. T. Thach. "Deaths and Near Deaths of Healthy Newborn Infants While Bed Sharing on Maternity Wards." *Journal of Perinatology* 34, no. 4 (2014): 275–79.

14. Sarah A. Keim, Joseph S. Hogan, Kelly A. McNamara, Vishnu Gudimetla, Chelsea E. Dillon, Jesse J. Kwiek, and Sheela R. Geraghty. "Microbial Contamination of Human Milk Purchased via the Internet." *Pediatrics* 132, no. 5 (2013): e1227–35.

CHAPTER 10. HOW NATURAL BIRTH IS ANTI-FEMINIST

1. C. K. Egbert. "Eve's Punishment Rebooted: The Ideology of Natural Birth." *Feminist Current*, July 3, 2014. Accessed April 18, 2015. %3A%2F%2Ffeministcurrent.com%2F9237%2Feves-punishment -rebooted-the-ideology-of-natural-birth%2F.

2. "The Caravan | The Farm Midwives." The Caravan | The Farm Midwives. Accessed January 26, 2016. http://www.thefarmmidwives.org /the_caravan.html.

3. "Bloomberg's Breastfeeding Program, 'Latch On NYC,' Wants Hospitals to Change Baby Formula Protocol." *The Huffington Post*, July 30, 2012. Accessed April 18, 2015. huffingtonpost.com/2012/07/30 /bloombergs-breast-feeding-latch-on-nyc-hospitals-hide-baby-for mula_n_1718664.html.

4. Betty Friedan. *The Feminine Mystique*, 20th anniversary edition. New York: Dell, 1983. Originally published in 1963.

5. Jennifer Schuessler. "Criticisms of a Classic Abound." *New York Times*. February 18, 2013. Accessed April 17, 2015. nytimes.com/2013/02 /19/books/50-years-of-reassessing-the-feminine-mystique.html ?_r=0.

6. "The Feminine Mystique." Wikipedia. Accessed April 17, 2015. en .wikipedia.org/wiki/The_Feminine_Mystique.

7. Sheila Kitzinger. "Why Feminists HATE Natural Childbirth . . . and

Why Their Prejudice Can Harm Mothers AND Their Babies, by the Woman Who Taught a Generation How to Give Birth." *Mail Online*. May 5, 2015. dailymail.co.uk/femail/article-3068100/Why-feminists -HATE-natural-childbirth-prejudice-harm-mothers-babies-woman -taught-generation-birth.html.

8. K. Beckett. "Choosing Cesarean: Feminism and the Politics of Childbirth in the United States." *Feminist Theory* 6, no. 3 (2005): 251–75.

9. "Idealized and Industrialized Labor: Anatomy of a Feminist Controversy." *Hypatia* 27, no. 1 (2012): 99–117.

10. Mariah Sixkiller. "Why I Am a Birth Feminist." *The Daily Beast*, July 26, 2015. Accessed December 2, 2015. thedailybeast.com/articles /2015/07/26/why-i-am-a-birth-feminist.html.

CHAPTER 11. WOMEN DO NOT HAVE OTHER WAYS OF KNOWING

1. Jane Munro and Helen Spiby. "The Nature and Use of Evidence in Midwifery Care," in *Evidence Based Midwifery: Applications in Context*, eds. Helen Spiby and Jane Munro. *Evidence Based Midwifery: Applications in Context*. New York: Wiley, 2009.

2. David L. Sackett, William Rosenberg, J. A. Gray, R. Brian Haynes, and W. Scott Richardson. "Evidence Based Medicine: What It Is and What It Isn't." *BMJ* 312, no. 7023 (1996): 71–72.

3. Sara Wickham. "Evidence-Informed Midwifery. 1. What Is Evidence-Informed Midwifery?" *Midwifery Today with International Midwife* 51 (1998): 42–43.

4. Marieke Saher and Marjaana Lindeman. "Alternative Medicine: A Psychological Perspective." *Personality and Individual Differences* 39, no. 6 (2005): 1169–78.

5. David G. Myers. *Intuition: Its Powers and Perils*. New Haven: Yale University Press, 2004.

6. Marjaana Lindeman and Kia Aarnio. "Superstitious, Magical, and Paranormal Beliefs: An Integrative Model." *Journal of Research in Personality* 41, no. 4 (2007): 731–44.

7. Ina May Gaskin. *Spiritual Midwifery*. Summertown, TN: Book Publications, 1997, p. 270.

8. Robbie Davis-Floyd. "Ways of Knowing: Open and Closed Systems." *Midwifery Today Int Midwife* 69 (2004): 9–13.

9. David Dunning. "We Are All Confident Idiots." *Pacific Standard Magazine*, October 27, 2014. Accessed April 18, 2015. psmag.com /health-and-behavior/confident-idiots-92793.

CHAPTER 12. SANCTIMOMMIES AND THE JOYS OF SHAMING

1. Rebecca Kukla. "Measuring Mothering." *International Journal of Feminist Approaches to Bioethics* 1, no. 1 (2008): 67–90.

2. J. Macvarish. "Effect of 'Risk-Thinking' on the Contemporary Construction of Teenage Motherhood." *Health, Risk and Society* 12, no. 4 (August 2010): 313–22. doi:10.1080/13698571003789724.

3. Candace Johnson. "The Political 'Nature' of Pregnancy and Childbirth." *Canadian Journal of Political Science* 41, no. 4 (2008): 889–913.

4. Arthur Chu. "Who Died and Made You Khaleesi?" *The Daily Beast*. June 24, 2014. Accessed April 18, 2015. thedailybeast.com/articles /2014/06/24/who-died-and-made-you-khaleesi-privilege-white-sav iors-and-the-elusive-male-feminist-who-doesn-t-suck.print.html.

5. "The Safe Motherhood Quilt Project." Remember the Mothers. Accessed April 18, 2015. rememberthemothers.org/.

6. Orit Avishai. "Managing the Lactating Body: The Breastfeeding Project in the Age of Anxiety," in *Infant Feeding Practices: A Cross-Cultural Perspective*, ed. Pranee Liamputtong. New York: Springer, 2011, pp. 23–38.

7. Jessica Martin-Weber. "The Romanticized Myth of What Constitutes Successful Breastfeeding: An Apology." *The Leaky Boob*, October 15, 2014. theleakyboob.com/2014/10/the-romanticized-myth-of-what -constitutes-successful-breastfeeding-an-apology/.

8. Norah MacKendrick. "More Work for Mother: Chemical Body Burdens as a Maternal Responsibility." *Gender & Society* 28, no. 5 (2014): 705–28.

Image Credits

Page 56 Courtesy of the author.

Page 58 Courtesy of the author.

Page 60 M. F. MacDorman, S. E. Kirmeyer, and E. C. Wilson. "Fetal and Perinatal Mortality, United States, 2006." *National Vital Statistics Reports from the Centers for Disease Control and Prevention*, National Center for Health Statistics, National Vital Statistics System 60, no. 8 (2012): 1–22.

Page 127 Courtesy of the author.

Page 128 Courtesy of the author.

Page 133 Cynthia G. Colen and David M. Ramey. "Is Breast Truly Best? Estimating the Effects of Breastfeeding on Long-Term Child Health and Wellbeing in the United States Using Sibling Comparisons." *Social Science & Medicine* 109 (2014): 55–65.

Page 195 Courtesy of the author.

Page 252 "Baby-Friendly USA, Inc. Fee Schedule." Baby-Friendly USA, Inc., May 1, 2014. Accessed April 18, 2015.

Index